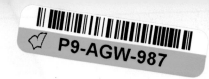

WIGS

Sally Cooney

and Charlotte Harper

WIGS

A Complete Guide
for the Profession

Illustrated by George Goode

Prentice-Hall, Englewood Cliffs, New Jersey

Library of Congress Cataloging in Publication Data

COONEY, SALLY
    Wigs; a complete guide for the profession.

    1. Wigs. I. Harper, Charlotte
joint author. II. Title.
TT975.C66   646.7'248   73-8417
ISBN 0-13-957761-0

Printed in the United States of America

10 9 8 7 6 5 4 3 2 1

Prentice-Hall International, Inc., London
Prentice-Hall of Australia, Pty. Ltd., Sydney
Prentice-Hall of Canada, Ltd., Toronto
Prentice-Hall of India Private Limited, New Delhi
Prentice-Hall of Japan, Inc., Tokyo

CONTENTS

WIGS

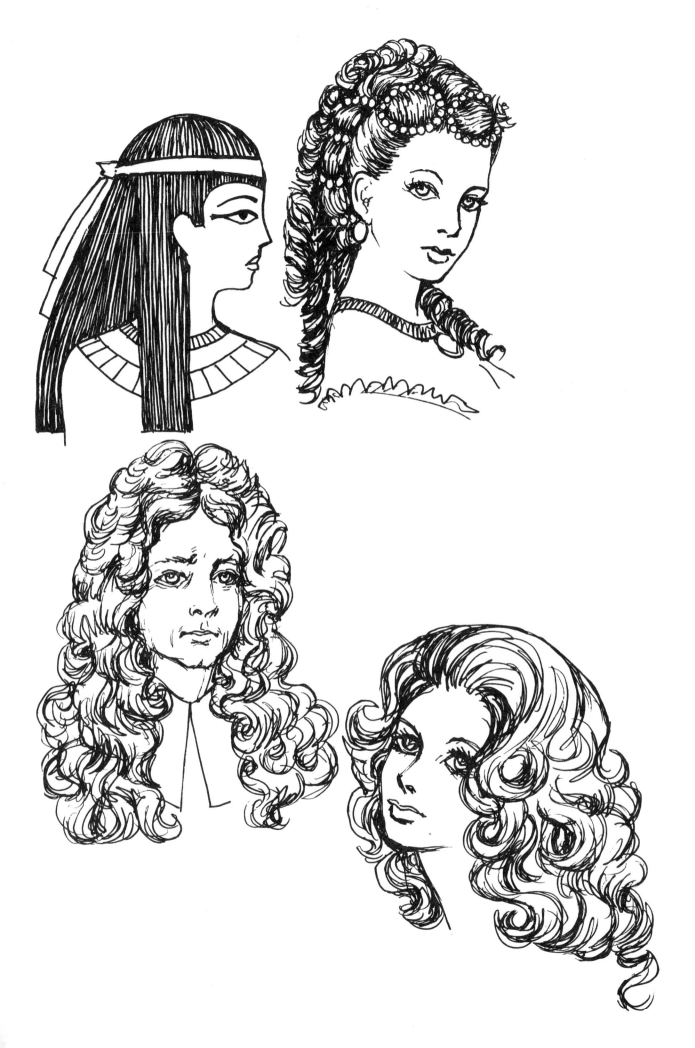

Chapter 1   HISTORY OF WIGS

WHAT IS A WIG?

A wig is an artificial head of hair or hairpiece worn as a personal or theatrical adornment, disguise, or, at one time, as a symbol of office. The word wig is the shortened form of periwig or peruke (French). The wearing of wigs by both sexes dates from the earliest recorded time. The wig "business" has been well established since 4000 B.C., when wigs were made of palm and wool fibers, animal hair, and even gold and silver metals. Both men and women in Egypt shaved their heads for religious customs and wore wigs for stature, beauty, and to keep their heads clean and free from vermin in the hot Egyptian climate.

In the beginning, wig-makers made no attempt to imitate natural hair. Wigs were decorative and often indicative of rank. The bigger the wig, the higher the official of state. These coifs went from braids to spiral curls, held tightly in place with the earliest affixative—bee's wax. The periwig of the sixteenth century merely simulated real hair, either as an adornment or to correct nature's defects. During the seventeenth century in France, the periwig was worn as a distinctive feature of costume. In 1624, Louis XIII, prematurely bald, also adopted one and thus set the fashion. After the restoration in England, under Charles II, the wearing of the peruke became general. Under Queen Anne the wig attained its maximum development, covering the back and shoulders and floating down over the chest.

1

Many varieties were perfected, the cheaper versions being of horse-hair. Smaller, less pretentious wigs, custom-ordered from London, were also worn in the American colonies. Women in general did not wear wigs but had their own hair (sometimes with the addition of false hair) elaborately dressed and powdered.

Wigs were differentiated according to class and professions. When early in the reign of George III, the general fashion of wearing wigs began to wane and die out, the practice held its own among professional men. Doctors, soldiers, and clergymen gave up the custom by slow degrees. In the church it survived longest among the bishops. Both the French and American Revolutions saw the sweeping away of many social customs, including class distinctions indicated by hair styles and wigs. Wigs are now worn as part of the official costume only in Great Britain by judges and barristers.

With the development of television and greater emphasis upon youthfulness, the ancient art of wig-making came full cycle. After the early 1950s the use of men's hairpieces, known as toupees, was increasingly accepted, and very convincing toupees, secure, yet undetectable, were developed. In the 1960s wigs for women again became fashionable, and many styles were designed to be undetectable. Additional hair pieces continued to be used to build up elaborate evening hair styles.

It has been said that blond hair is worth its weight in gold. At one time the main source was Northern Italy, where girls may still sell their hair to provide a dowry. Coarser hair from Japan and Korea was less costly but did not hold a set as well. Nylon and other synthetic hair was used especially for inexpensive costume styles. Anywhere from 50,000 to 300,000 strands of hair are used in a full-head wig, which is made by knotting each hair by hand, by the end that was cut from the head so that it will actually appear to be growing and will brush naturally, on to a cotton, or silk foundation. Less expensive wigs were made by sewing small bundles of human, synthetic, or goat hair onto a canvas cap, by hand or machine.

There have been vast changes in the wig business of today. Raw hair can be processed to a finer texture than the natural hair. The improvement in processing has made all the wigs on today's market much better than those produced even ten years ago. European hair is considered the best quality, but the better manufacturers of Oriental hair have made their products comparable for a much lower cost. The synthetic has been upgraded to a more manageable fiber that looks and acts more like human hair.

WHY WOMEN WEAR WIGS

Women wear wigs for many reasons: for adornment and convenience, and to correct nature's faults. Wigs can give a person a variety of hair styles to complement any fashion, occasion, or outing. An elaborate style, suitable for evening wear can be obtained in a moment with the putting on of a pre-styled wig over one's own hair, or, a casual style may be worn over a pin-curled hair set, while a woman does her shopping. In addition, wigs are a perfect cover-up after swimming. Hair pieces and falls give added body to the thin-haired woman, and wigs are worn by women who have lost hair due to treatments of chemical therapy or surgery.

IDENTIFICATION OF WIGS AND HAIRPIECES

There are several kinds of wigs and hair pieces available in many types of hair and fiber. Some are hand-tied, some are machine-made, and others are made partially by machine and partially by hand. Here, we will outline the different kinds of hair pieces, learn to identify them, and suggest some styles for the individual pieces. Learn your merchandise and what it can do.

Identifying Types of Wigs

The *hand-tied* wig cap is made entirely of a lightweight mesh, usually of silk or nylon. Strands, containing from five to eight individual hairs, are looped around and through the mesh of the cap where they are tied and tightened down to the cap. This construction is easily identifiable by holding the wig up to the light and looking through the inside of the cap. The mesh and individual strands can easily be distinguished.

The *machine-made* wig caps are usually of cotton or nylon mesh, much heavier than the silk type used for hand-tied wigs. Hair strands are machine-sewn into strips or wefts of hair (refer to drawings on page 9). These wefts are then machine-sewn onto caps in horizontal rows from ear to ear. (An earlier method of applying the wefts to the cap was to sew them in a continuous circling pattern around the circumference of the cap coming to a point at the crown.) Today, further improvements have been made by machine-sewing a weft of hair around the inside perimeter of the cap so that when this hair is brushed out and back into the rest of the hair, the edge of the wig cap is hidden.

On the *semi-machine-made* wig, the outer section is hand-tied completely around the frame, then wefts are sewn onto the remainder of the cap. On hairpieces, the front section, approximately one-sixteenth of an inch back, is hand-tied. The remainder of the wig or hairpiece is machine wefts of hair sewn horizontally. The advantages and disadvantages of each type of wig are discussed under the heading "Quality Of Wigs," on page 8.

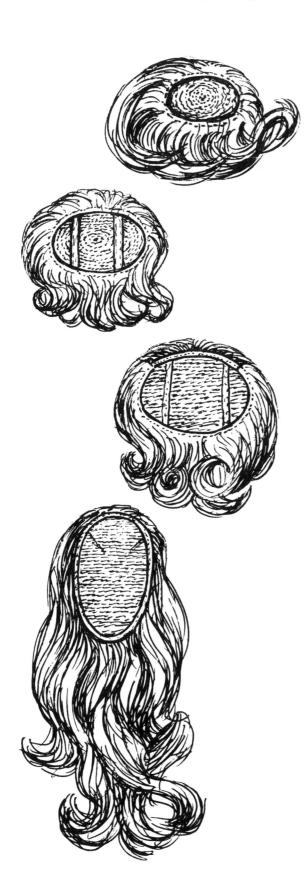

"SILVER DOLLAR" HAIR PIECE

How to distinguish:
Machine-made.
Small "silver dollar" base.
6 to 8 inches long.

Style suggestions:
Mostly designed for filler

HAIRPIECE WITH 3 INCH BASE

How to distinguish:
Machine made.
3 inch base.
6 to 8 inches long.

Style suggestions:
Filler
Curls

HAIRPIECE WITH HAND-TIED FRONT

How to distinguish:
Front-rim hair is tied by hand.
3 inch base.
10 to 12 inches long.

Style suggestions:
Long filler (put into short flips)
Curls

CASCADE HAIRPIECE

How to distinguish:
Machine-made (some with hand-tied front).
Oblong base approximately 5 inches long and 2 inches wide at top, base narrowing to 1½ inches at bottom.
10 to 12 inches long.

Style suggestions:
Curls
Buns
Braided
Fillers

TOPETTE HAIRPIECE

How to distinguish:
Machine-made
(some with hand-tied front).
Large round base with 4 to 5 inch
diameter.
6 to 8 inches long.

Style suggestions:
Full coverage cap style for short
hair
Curls

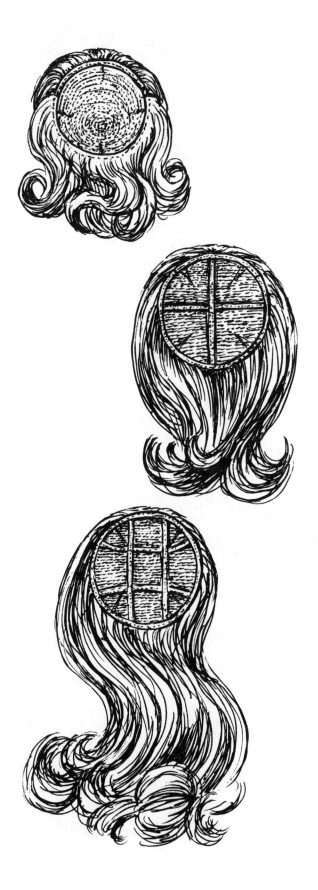

SHORT FALL
(often called a mini-fall)

How to distinguish:
Semi-machine-made.
4 to 5 inch diameter base.
12 to 14 inches long.
Weighs 5 to 6½ ounces.

Style suggestions:
Curls
Pageboy
Swing
Short flips

MEDIUM FALL
(often called midi-fall)

How to distinguish:
Semi-machine made.
4 to 5½ inch diameter base.
15 to 20 inches long.
Weighs 7 to 7½ ounces.

Style suggestions:
Flips
Long pageboy
Ponytails
Curls

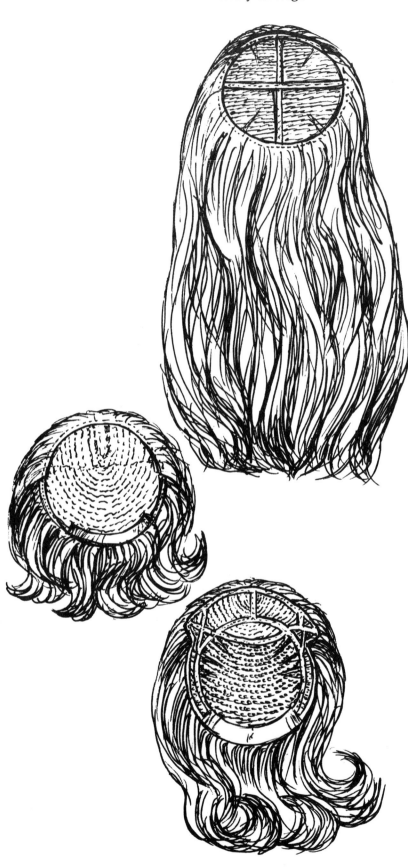

LONG FALL
(often called maxi-fall)

How to distinguish:
Semi-machine made.
4 to 6 inch diameter base.
20 to 26 inches long.
Weighs 8½ to 10 ounces.

Style suggestions:
Long soft flip
Loose curl
Double ponytail

MACHINE-MADE WIG

How to distinguish:
Entire wig is machine-sewn wefts
sewn circularly on cotton cap.
Weft of hair inside cap is machine
sewn.
Normal 22-inch cap size.
6 to 8 inches long.

Style suggestions:
Any shorter hair style desired for
full coverage

SEMI-MACHINE-MADE WIG

How to distinguish:
Hand-tied hair around complete
cap base.
Horizontal wefts machine-sewn
on remaining cap.
Normal 22 inch cap size.
Hair lengths: 10 to 12 inches, 12 to
15 inches, 24 inches, 36 inches.

Style suggestions:
Good for swept back style or bang
fronts
Shoulder flips
Pageboy
No style limitation

HAND-TIED WIG

How to distinguish:
No machine stitching.
Hair is hand-knotted to open-mesh cap.
Approximately 8 to 10 strands per knot in back and 6 to 8 strands in closer mesh of front frame of cap.
Hair lengths: 10 to 12 inches, 12 to 15 inches, 24 inches, 36 inches.

Styles:
Designed to look just like your favorite hairdo, there are no style limitations

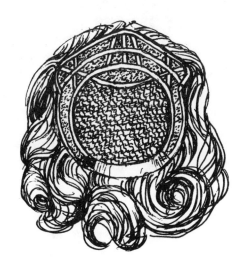

EUROPEAN WIG OR ORIENTAL WIG

How to distinguish:
By federal law, all wigs must be labeled as to the kind of hair, where and how made.

SYNTHETIC WIG
(made of Dynel, Kanekalon, Alura, Venicelon)

How to distinguish:
The match test is about the only sure way of telling if the hair is human or synthetic. Human hair will singe and form into small balls; synthetic fiber will melt from the heat and completely disintegrate.
Any length (pre-cut for specific style).

Styles:
Never needs set. Comb out in curls, fillers or any style suited to your customer's likes.

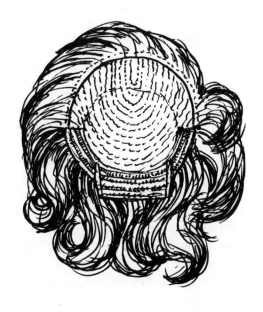

QUALITY OF WIGS

We have identified some of the more popular wigs, but now we need to consider the differences in the qualities of the different types of hair goods. Quality of wig hair is placed in two important groups before it is re-graded:

First-quality hair: cut from the head

Second-quality hair: obtained from combings and not cut directly from the head

Texture, porosity, elasticity *after* processing again categorizes the quality of hair used and the price structure for same.

Hand-made Wigs

The European hand-made wig is the finest quality wig on the market. The hair comes from the European countries where the hair is generally light in color and fine in texture, usually uncolored, with no permanent curl added to the hair, brushed to clean, and the best of care taken during the growth of the hair. These markets are located in France, Germany, and Italy, although the hair comes from all parts of Europe. European-hair wigs are not made of virgin hair. All hair is treated the same in processing, but European hair is better, healthier hair to start with. (For a full discussion of processing, see Chapter 8.) In all hand-made European wigs, there is absolutely no machine stitching; even the binding tapes are hand-stitched. The wig is labelled 100 percent human, European hair, hand-made. Because of the fine texture of the hair, the lightweight materials, such as pure silk, used in making the cap, and the fact that the wigs are entirely hand-made, the weight of this wig is light, between three and five ounces. Thus, the European wig is the most comfortable to wear, the prettiest to style, and the coolest. The cost of this type of merchandise to the buyer is high, but well worth it.

European Hair Wiglets and Falls

European hair wiglets and falls are the finest to have. Their quality is good, and their price high. Actually there is more hair in these pieces than in those of lesser quality, even though the entire weight is less. Falls do not even need teasing if a casual style is to be worn. The falls and wiglets are natural in appearance and comfortable to wear. The hair is so fine in texture that repeated styling with heavy teasing will ruin this piece, so European hair should be used to create a more natural effect. These, again, are like fine diamonds and should be treated as such.

Semi-machine-made Wigs

The semi-machine-made wig has a hand-tied front section and a machine-tied base from the front section to the back of the wig. In the machine-tied section, the hair is sewn on a weft and then sewn on to the cap.

EXAMPLE
Weft of hair

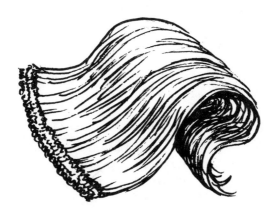

The hand-tied section generally runs entirely around the cap, from front to back. The foundation is generally made of cotton which is cool and easy to size, and lighter on the head than nylon. This type of wig is easily styled because the front section can go either forward or back, or the customer's hair can be blended into the front. This is one of the most popular, moderate-priced wigs on the market today, and the one you probably will sell more than any other.

Machine-made Wigs

The machine-made wig is of lesser quality and price. The styling of this wig has less potential than the semi-machine-made wig. It has a heavier cap, shorter lengths of hair, and machine wefts sewn in a circle onto the entire cap, usually ending in a ponytail in the center crown.

Synthetics

Synthetic wigs are sewn on a stretch base made of a reinforced elastic. They are generally machine-made. Some have handmade fronts, some have scalp parts, some are all hand-tied. The fiber sewn on wefts is pre-cut and sewn to create a particular style. A few of the better fibers are Alura by Monsanto, Dynel produced by Union Carbide, and Venice-lon, an Italian fiber.

The principle of the synthetic is that the wig is bought for its style and should never have to be rolled. The customer can wash this wig for herself. The synthetic wig is great for casual wear and will withstand damp or wet weather.

Oriental Hand-made

As the name of this wig type states, it is of Oriental origin, made in China, Korea, or Japan. For some time now the better made of this category have been made in Hong Kong, China, and most recently Korea. This wig is, of course, labeled by law. When you examine the inner cap you will see the binding in the cap has been machine-sewn together, although the rest of the hair has been tied onto the cap. Oriental hair of good processing has been found to be very good and of lasting quality.

Oriental hair is strong and with modern processing is almost as fine in texture as European hair. This hair ranges from dark brown to black in color. The hand-tied Oriental wig is lighter in weight, cooler, and easier to style than a machine-made wig. One point that should be made of hand-tied wigs is the fact that they are more delicate than machine-made wigs and should be cared for in a more gentle manner. With proper care, they will give several years of service.

Hairpieces

Hairpieces are additional, add-in, pieces that constitute a part of a hairstyle. The most common hairpiece is totally machine-sewn. (See the diagram under Machine-made Wigs, p. 6.) Semi-machine-made hairpieces have a front section of hair hand knotted. The base of this hairpiece will fit much closer to the head and pin in more easily, since the base is not as thick. Some cascades have handtied fronts; the most commonly used is all machine-made with a bound edge. Most falls have a hand-tied front section, since they were designed to comb back with the customer's hair combed over the front. Base sizes and lengths of hair vary from mini to the maxi lengths.

EXERCISE

1. How long has the wig business been in existence?

_____

2. What were the first wigs made of? _____

3. List at least five reasons a person would be interested in any additional hair.

A. _____   B. _____   C. _____   D. _____   E. _____

4. Give one use for each:

Hand-tied wig: _____

Man-made wig: _____

Mini-fall: _____

Midi-fall: _____

Maxi-fall: _____

Toppette: _____

Cascade: _____

Hairpiece, flat base: _____

Alura: _____

5. What is a weft of hair? _____

6. What is first-quality hair? _____

7. What is second-quality hair? _____

8. Give the approximate weight of a European hand-tied wig.

_____

9. What is an Oriental wig? _____

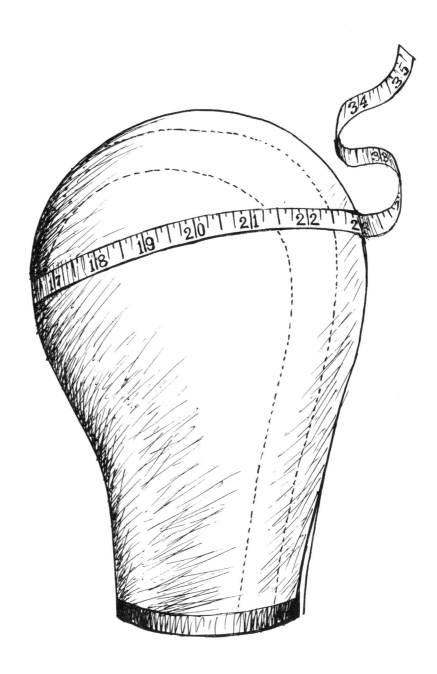

Chapter 2

SIZING AND BLOCKING

WIG SIZING

There have been millions of wigs sold in this country in the last few years. These wigs have been sold with the promise that they will solve the hair problems that the customers have. There is one important question you must consider when you sell a wig and that is, will it fit? If the wig does not fit, it will be unstylable and almost unwearable. This is where your knowledge of sizing will come in. You can take any wig (the standard size of a wig cap is about 22 inches around) and make it fit any head from an 18 to a 24 if you know your merchandise and how to size it. For example: A cotton cap of size 22 will stretch to a 24 by wetting it with hot water and stretching on to a 24-inch block, but a wig made with a nylon cap will not stretch. A cotton cap will shrink to a certain degree and retain its size without darting, whereas a nylon cap will not.

In the sizing chapter we will teach you how to cut a wig, dart it, stretch, shrink, and repair it. The sizing is basic to all of your work. If a wig is baggy in the crown on the block, it stands to reason that when you cut the wig and it is placed on the customer's head, although the bagginess is pulled out by the fullness of her crown, the wig will have a gap; this will not be due to a deficiency in your cutting ability, but because you have failed to block the wig properly according to your customer's head size. If the wig is too low over the ears, the wig will be too long, and if you then take up the wig on the inside of the cap, the wig may then be too short if it has been previously cut, so you must measure carefully before you ever start to cut and style a wig.

Some of the things that can be done to a wig to alter its size and fit are: cut it apart and then sew it back together reducing the size by cutting the material down; replace the elastic; sew up or darn the holes; stretch it; add hair; cut the back out to expose the customer's hair in back.

Most of this work is considered custom work. There is not anything you, as a professional, cannot do to a wig to fit it, as long as you know what you are doing, and this is exactly what we want to teach you in this chapter.

CONSTRUCTION OF WIG CAP

The sizing and blocking of wigs is as important as the style. A proper fit is essential, not only for appearance, but for the comfort of the wearer.

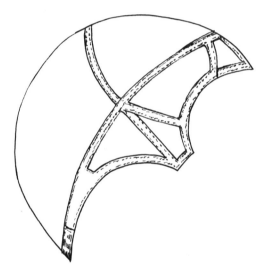

STEP 1: SIZING

Brush the customer's hair back from face and neck, and secure it in place by pinning the bulk of it at the crown. If the hair is long it should be divided and pinned securely and flat at center crown.

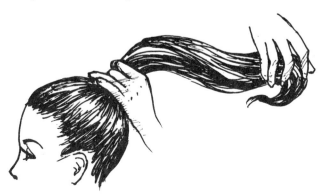

Twist the base and wind the hair into a coil. Place into a flat chignon and secure with bobby pins.

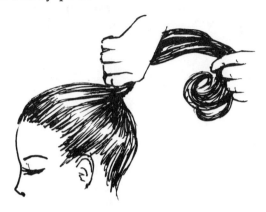

The head is now ready to receive the wig. Note the smooth distribution of hair, creating height where needed.

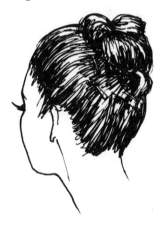

STEP 2: WIG MEASUREMENT INSTRUCTIONS

FIRST MEASUREMENT AROUND HEAD: Make sure tape is behind ears and follows hairline. Start tape at center front hairline, continue it around, ending at the center front.

SECOND MEASUREMENT EAR TO EAR: Measure across front hairline from ear to ear with one-half inch between ear and tape. Take tape over top of the head about two inches behind the hairline.

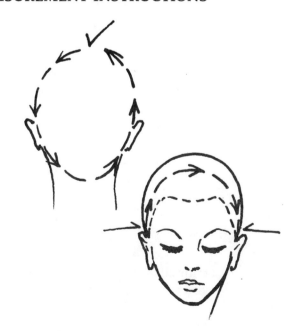

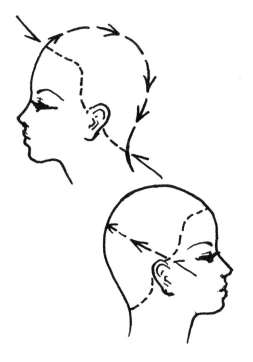

THIRD MEASUREMENT FRONT TO BACK: Measure from widow's peak, to base of the skull at the occipital bone, over top of head.

FOURTH MEASUREMENT TEMPLE TO TEMPLE: Place tape on temple side, held by the thumb, and measure around back crown of head to left temple.

Always keep a card file on your customer with her completed measurements.

EXAMPLE:

NAME_____	PHONE	Home_____
		Office_____
ADDRESS_____		
CITY_____	STATE_____	ZIP_____
HEAD MEASUREMENTS	Hair piece: (kind)	
Around the head:	Hair sample:	
Ear to ear:	Date:	
Front to back:	Style:	
Temple to temple:		

Make this card a part of your permanent record.

NOTE—SALES HELP: Always take the card from your files when your customer brings her wig to you. Not only does this remind her that you are equipped for her work, but it also helps create a professional attitude between you and your customer. You may ask her, "Shall we create a new style for you this week, perhaps a curly look, or do you prefer the same smooth full lines with the flip?"

ALTERATIONS

Sizing of New Wigs and Unsized Wigs

Select a canvas block the same size as your customer's head. Note: Do not go by the size on the block, but take a tape measure and measure around the largest part of the block. Most canvas blocks are filled with cork and will swell during regular salon use.

EXAMPLE:

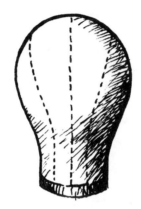

First, measure around the largest part of the block:

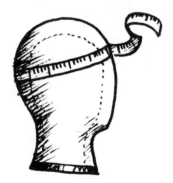

Pin off the customer's measurement, according to the card.

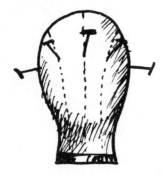
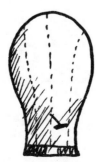

Now turn the wig wrong side out, and pin it to the block according to where you have placed the tee pins, keeping hair smooth inside the wig.

Slowly and gently work the bulk out of the wig. If the wig does not adhere to the measurements it can be made to fit either by darts or by "cutting-down," whichever is more appropriate in your customer's case.

For example:

THE LONG-HAIRED CUSTOMER.   When you measured your customer for the wig, you pinned the bulk of her hair to the crown section; thus her hair added to the measurements so no extra allowance needs to be made here. The only reason you would ever have to re-size her wig is if she cuts her hair.

THE SHORT-HAIRED CUSTOMER.   If your customer has short hair and intends to let it grow long, then you know it is best to dart the wig and not to cut it down. In six months or so you will have to let the darts out in the crown to make allowances for the longer hair.

THE THIN-HAIRED OR BALD.   Extra bulk in the wig of a customer who has lost her hair for some reason or another or who has very thin hair is unwarranted. The bulk should be cut out, to assure a closer to the head fit.

Darts

Darts are always taken so that the dart is inside the wig. Note: If you turn the dart the other way you will produce bulk in the outside of the wig and it will interfere with both style and cut. Make the dart and then baste it down with regular needle and fine upholstery thread. Use thread the color of the interior of the wig being sized. Horizontal tucks shorten the wig from front to back. Vertical tucks will make the wig shorter from ear to ear.

EXAMPLE 1   EXAMPLE 2

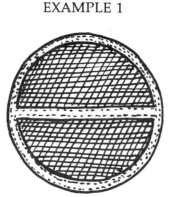
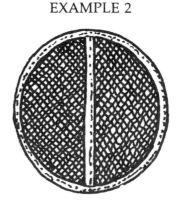

Horizontal tuck   Vertical tuck

Remember, if the wig fits too long from the front to the back you will tuck it horizontally, and if it is too deep over the ears you will make a vertical dart. The horizontal tuck should be done with a basting stitch and then whipped down, with the tuck always on the inside of the cap. Usually this is best done in the crown. The vertical tuck is done as the horizontal tuck except that you start at the nape of the neck.

Cutting Down Wigs

Most of the time when you cut a wig down, you cut it at the seam where the wig has been put together in the first place (see Examples 1 and 2). Do not be afraid to cut a wig if necessary; it can be put back together.

DRAWING OF WIG CAP

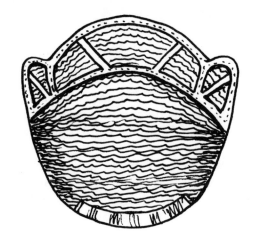

Stretching Wigs

If a wig is too small for the customer, the same sizing technique is used, except that in order to stretch a wig on the block you must turn it wrong side out, wet the inside of the cap, and slowly stretch the wig to the measurements you have pinned off on the block. Stretch the wig with a slow kneading type of pressure to insure complete stretching of wig. Uneven pressure in any one area may cause ripping. Once you have stretched the wig it will stay if the wig is always put on the right size of block.

Now that you have sized the wig there is only one more step. In the back of most wigs there is an elastic band. This elastic should be pulled to fit the block to which you have sized your customer's wig, and then pinned with a small gold safety pin. Note: Do not tie or knot the elastic. The pin is used in place of stitching because the elastic will stretch over a period of time and it may need to be re-adjusted. Heat of the head will relax the elastic, and cleaning fluids will deteriorate it. On the other hand, if the wig is a little too tight, the elastic can be easily let out by moving the pin.

Once or twice a year you will need to replace a worn-out elastic. First, loosen the stitches at the beginning, or place where the elastic is sewn down, and then pull the elastic out of the free end. Place a small gold safety pin on the end of the new elastic and then run it back through where you took it out. Make a small incision in the sewn-down end and pull the small gold safety pin through. Then stitch down the elastic, darn where you cut, and pin the free end.

EXAMPLE OF ELASTIC

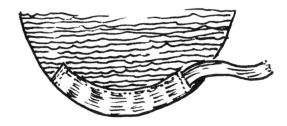

Blocking

Blocking hair pieces, falls, and other smaller pieces of hair is most important. Place the piece on the canvas head at the place it is to fit on the customer's head, so that the stylist can balance the piece in combing it.

When you place the tee pins in any hairpiece, be sure that you pin it at an angle, otherwise when you comb, the piece will pull off the block. It takes only four tee pins to hold a hair piece, and six to hold a fall, on the block.

To pin a wig on the block properly, use six tee pins, one at each ear section, one at the center front, one at center back and one behind each ear. You must again angle these tee pins to avoid pulling the wig off the block while combing it.

EXAMPLE

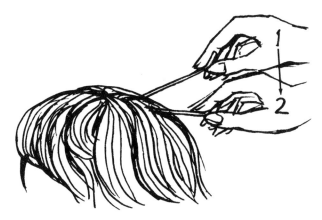

Hold tee pins at a 45° angle, push through the hairpiece only, turn down to a horizontal angle, and push into the block.

EQUIPMENT USED IN SIZING AND BLOCKING

Tape measure   Vice or clamp
Index cards   Needle and thread
Canvas block   Scissors (not hair cutting
Tee pins   scissors)
                             Gold safety pins

EXERCISE

1. Describe the four most important measurements for a customer's head size.

A. _____   B. _____   C. _____

D. _____

2. After a wig is sized, is this a permanent thing?

_____

3. How are customers' measurements transferred to wig block?

_____

4. How is a wig placed on block to transfer block measurements to cap?

_____

5. When should a cap be cut down instead of darting?

_____

6. What color thread should be used on a wig being sized?

_____

7. Why are cap sizes so important?_____

8. Should a wig be cut before it is sized? Why?

_____

9. If your customer has short hair when a wig is sized, can it be re-sized if her hair grows long? _____

10. How many tee pins does it normally take to block a wig?_____

11. Does it matter where a hairpiece, fall, etc. is pinned to the block?

_____

12. List eight pieces of equipment used in sizing and blocking.

A. _____   E. _____

B. _____   F. _____

C. _____   G. _____

D. _____   H. _____

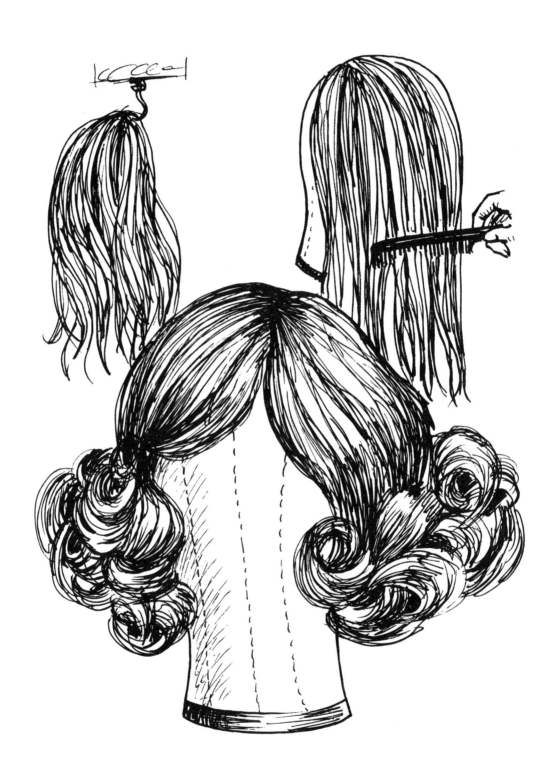

Chapter 3   CLEANING AND CONDITIONING

Like any piece of clothing we put on our body, wigs should be kept clean. A wig will lose its luster, softness, and manageability when it is dirty. All *new* wigs must be cleaned and some conditioned to protect the customer from any previous handling and from protective sprays used in shipping. In use, a wig will absorb cooking, smoking, and hair oil secretion odors. If a wig is worn on the average of once or twice a week, a person should have it cleaned every six to eight weeks. If a wig is worn every day, it should be cleaned every two weeks. This will protect the wig and keep the hair soft and manageable. These times are average; some people will need their wigs cleaned more frequently.

CLEANING A MACHINE-MADE HUMAN HAIR WIG

Brushing

First brush the hair to remove all spray, teasing, and tangles. Starting with the back of the wig, brush from the end of the hair all the way into the cap, until all teasing is out in this section, working up to the crown. Next, beginning at the sides of the wig by the ears, brush from the ends of the hair into cap again until all teasing is eliminated, working up to crown on both sides. Then start at the bang area, brushing the ends of the hair first, working into base until all teasing is removed. Work back to crown. A machine-made wig may be cleaned off the block.

EXAMPLE:

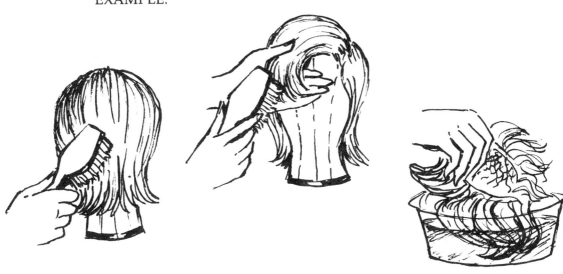

Cleaning

In a glass or porcelain bowl, place enough liquid dry-cleaning fluid to immerse the entire wig. Be sure to wear gloves to protect your hands. Put the hair in first until the solution covers the wig cap. With a small, soft brush, such as a manicure brush or a soft toothbrush, gently rub the inside of the front of the cap from ear to ear, across the front of the cap, removing all makeup and hair oil. Soak the wig for three to four minutes. Using a wide-tooth comb, comb through the hair, making sure all hair spray and oil is cleaned out. From the cap base to the ends of the hair, work your fingers through the hair to make sure the cleaning fluid goes throughout the wig. Squeeze excess fluid out of the wig. Towel blot, hang over bowl, and let drip dry. The drying process will take about 30 minutes. Brush the hair, and block according to customer's size. Spray the hair with water or immerse in water. If conditioner is to be used, apply the conditioner, and cover the wig with a plastic cap for 20 to 30 minutes. At the end of this time, remove the plastic cap, and with the wig still on the block, rinse it with water, comb with a wide-tooth comb, and set the style. To use an *instant* conditioner, first, spray the wig with water until wet, comb smooth with a wide-tooth comb, and blot with towel. Apply the instant conditioner, comb it through the wig, and then set.

All human hair pieces, cascades, and falls, should be cleaned in this manner.

EXAMPLE:

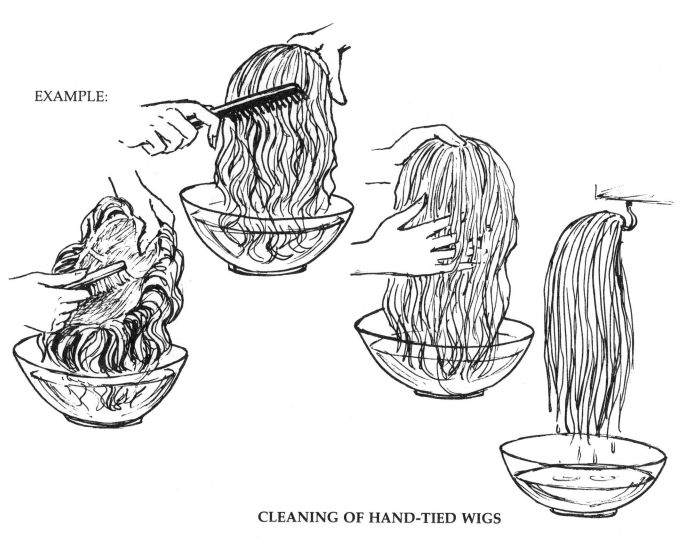

CLEANING OF HAND-TIED WIGS

Delicate hand-tied wigs should be cleaned on the block. Wrap plastic wrap around the canvas block. Before blocking, clean the inside of the cap with a brush. Block the wig. Immerse it in solution, let soak three to four minutes, and comb the solution through the wig hair. Work the solution from base to ends of hair with fingers. Towel blot. Allow to dry 20 to 30 minutes. Spray until wet, condition if necessary, and set.

EXAMPLE:

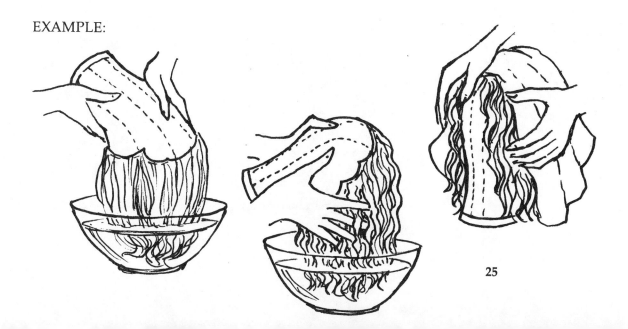

25

CLEANING INSTRUCTIONS FOR SYNTHETIC WIGS

Brush all teasing from the wig, loosening as much spray net as possible. Work the brush from the ends of the fiber into the base, so as not to break or tear the fiber loose from the cap. After all teasing is removed, the wig should not be brushed or combed again until after it has been washed and is completely dry. Fiber will stretch while wet, and the curl in the synthetic hair can be destroyed by combing the fiber when it is wet.

Place the wig shampoo (which must be mild, such as baby shampoo or special wig shampoo) in a glass bowl, deep enough to immerse entire wig. Use tepid to cool water; hot water will very often remove the curl. Using your fingers, work the suds through the fiber and the entire cap, being sure all makeup traces are removed from the cap and the hair around the ears. Beginning at one ear, work across the front of the cap to the other ear section. Rinse several times in tepid to cool water. DO NOT USE HOT WATER. When the rinse water is clear, *squeeze* all excess water from the wig. Do not twist or wring water out of the wig. Towel blot. Place the wig on a towel to dry, preferably with the cap turned to the outside for the first few hours of drying time. Do *not* place the wet wig on a block to dry. Drying on blocks will set the size of the stretch base and change the fit of your customer's wig. Wigs may be pinned up by the back hair and allowed to drip dry; they will dry faster in this manner because of the air circulation. It will take from five to twelve hours for the cap to dry completely. When it is dry, brush the hair, and spray it lightly with lanolin spray. The lanolin will give more luster and will keep the fiber from becoming dry-looking. The wig is now ready for combing. If shorter drying time is necessary, the wig may be placed in a cool dryer with only the fan blowing.

EXAMPLE:

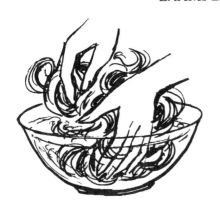
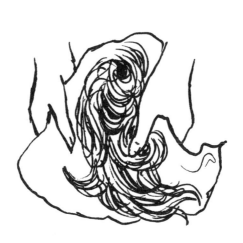
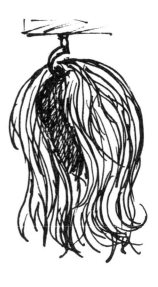

EQUIPMENT USED IN CLEANING AND CONDITIONING

Dry cleaning solution,
   for human hair only

Conditioners and instant
   conditioners

Deep glass or porcelain
   bowl

Wig shampoo or baby
   shampoo

Large-tooth comb

Small brush, such as a
   manicure brush, for
   inside of wig

Rubber gloves

EXERCISE

1. When should a wig be cleaned? _____

   _____

2. Must a human hair, machine-made wig be cleaned on a block?

   _____

3. What are the basic cleaning instructions for a machine-made wig?

   _____

4. What are the basic cleaning instructions for a human-hair, hand-tied

   wig? _____

5. What pieces require special cleaning? _____

6. What are the basic cleaning instructions for a synthetic wig? _____

   _____

7. List the equipment needed for cleaning and conditioning:

   A. _____

   B. _____

   C. _____

   D. _____

   E. _____

   F. _____

   G. _____

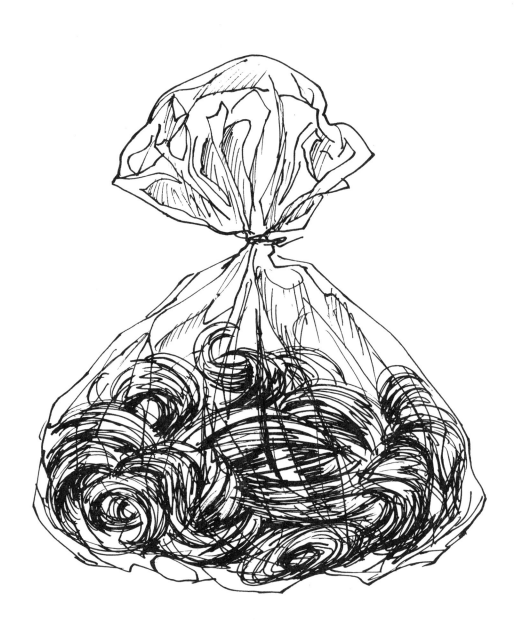

Chapter 4 SANITATION AND STERILIZATION

Sanitation and sterilization are important in the wig business because your customer is leaving a part of her wardrobe in your custody, and it is expected of you to protect her health and well-being as you would your own. We must understand the spread and control of disease in handling other people's hairgoods. Cleanliness and sanitation are the most important factors in our business since we are serving the public.

Bacteria, the microscopic vegetable organisms that cause disease, are found everywhere.

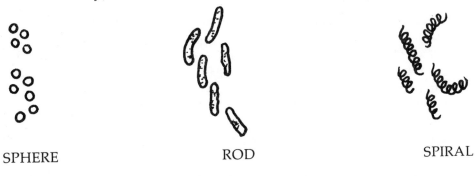

SPHERE   ROD   SPIRAL

BACTERIA

They are not visible to the naked eye, and hundreds of bacteria can be present and still not be seen. Head lice, small, wingless creatures with flat, almost transparent bodies, should be checked for on wig caps, particularly in the seams.

HEAD LOUSE

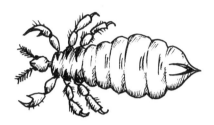

Steaming or boiling is necessary to destroy lice; physicians often prescribe a wash with a solution of benzyl benzoate to kill lice.

Wigs being an item of clothing able to foster bacteria, it is important to understand sanitization and sterilization as they apply to our business. Sterilization prevents the growth of germs. Some methods of sterilization are:

Boiling in water (at 212° Fahrenheit for 20 minutes)

Steaming (used mainly by the medical field to sterilize their instruments)

Dry heat (used to sterilize towels, sheets, cotton, gauze, etc.)

Ultraviolet rays (produced by an electric sanitizer and easily used in our business)

Antiseptics and disinfectants (a chemical agent used on combs, brushes, and all metal instruments)

Fumigants (a chemical vapor used in cabinets where combs, brushes, and other equipment are stored until used)

HOW TO CLEAN YOUR COMBS AND BRUSHES

Always remove all hair from combs and brushes before washing. Wash them in hot, soapy water, immerse in a disinfectant, and rinse thoroughly. The immersion of implements in a chemical solution should conform to the State Board regulations issued by your state. Place the combs and brushes in a cabinet with ultraviolet rays, and then store them in a drawer or cabinet with a fumigant until ready for use.

SANITARY BUSINESS PRACTICES

To help insure the health of your customers when wigs, hairpieces, or other hair is brought into your salon for service, place each item of hair in a separate "baggie" (plastic bag with fold-over top) and tag it with instructions listing all work required, before placing it in the appropriate bin for the service day requested.

Do not be afraid to *refuse* service on an item that needs cleaning if the customer does not want to go to the expense of cleaning it. First, it is unsanitary not to clean it. Second, the hair will not style well without proper cleaning, and *you* will get the blame for it.

Cleaning Equipment and Work Areas

Fumigants should be kept in all bins holding customer service pieces. All canvas blocks must be cleaned with an antiseptic before and after use with each customer piece. Tee pins should be cleaned with a solution of 70 percent alcohol. Any that show signs of rust must be discarded. All cutting implements are best sanitized with 70 percent alcohol.

Floors, sinks, and toilet bowls in a wig salon should be disinfected with Lysol, Pine Sol, or some similar disinfectant. Deodorizers are useful, too, in offsetting any offensive odors. Floors and stations must be cleaned after customers to insure cleanliness for your next customer.

The use of chemical agents can involve certain dangers. To insure safety, always follow these procedures:

1. Purchase all chemicals in small quantities.
2. Store all chemicals in a cool, dry area.
3. Label all containers.
4. Read and follow all instructions for mixing recommended by manufacturer.

The professional equipment used in sanitation and sterilization of your salon and equipment includes:

PROFESSIONAL EQUIPMENT

Ster-O-Matic
(Wet & Dry)

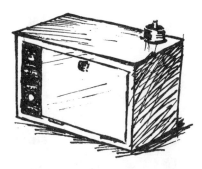

Dry Ster-O-Matic

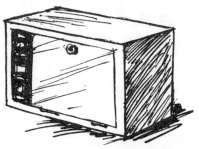

Air Purifier

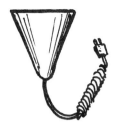

Brush & Comb Cleaner

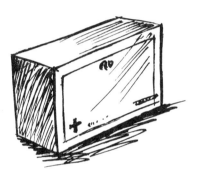

Sanitizer

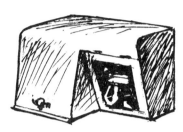

Taking care of your customers starts with sanitation and sterilization of your salon. Without a healthy customer, you do not have a business. If you take care of her, she, in turn, will bring you more business. This is our objective, and one never to make light of.

EXERCISE

1. Why should you practice sanitation and sterilization? _____

   _____

2. Define bacteria. _____

3. What will destroy bacteria? _____

4. At what degree Fahrenheit must water be to boil? _____
   How long should one boil an item to disinfect it?_____

5. What is a fumigant? _____

6. What is a disinfectant? _____

7. How should combs and brushes be sanitized? _____

   _____

8. Where should you store sanitized combs and brushes? _____

   _____

9. What do physicians prescribe to kill head lice? _____

10. Why should wigs be cleaned? _____

11. How do you clean a canvas block? _____

12. What should be done with tee pins that show signs of rust? _____

13. How can tee pins be cleaned? _____

14. With what should cutting implements be cleaned? _____

    _____

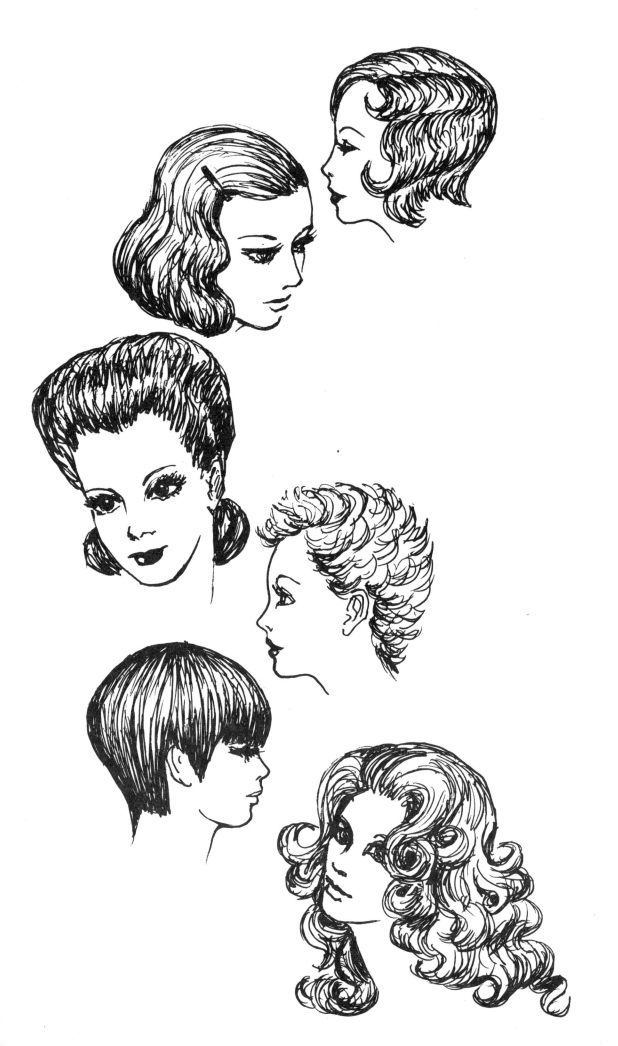

Chapter 5

HAIR CUTTING

Never cut a wig that does not fit; to cut a wig that does not fit is no better than not cutting the wig at all. Most haircutting problems on wigs come from the fact that the wig has not been properly sized for the individual to start with. A wig is a very personal thing and should be treated with respect. A style cannot be accomplished without a good basic cut; a good basic cut cannot be accomplished without first sizing the wig; and a wig cannot be sized until an individual says, "Yes, I want this wig. The color and texture are right for me, and the lengths of hair are right for the cut I want on my wig." This can be the beginning of a "beautiful relationship" between owner and wig. Now the rest is up to us. The art of haircutting on a wig should not be skimmed over; it takes much study and practice. The very basis of a pretty coiffed wig is the way you cut and fit the piece.

The style must contour to the patron's own personality and social activities.

Implements Needed

1. Regular hair shaping scissors

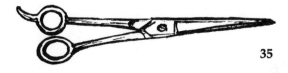

2. Thinning shears

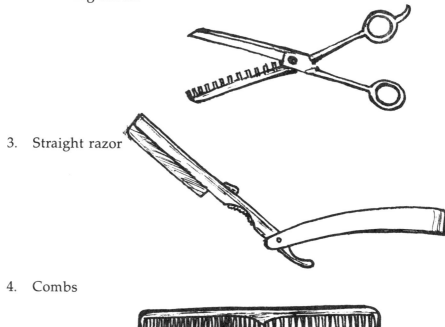

3. Straight razor

4. Combs

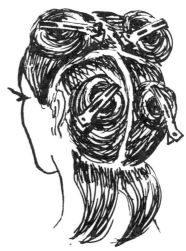

SECTIONING THE HAIR FOR SHAPING

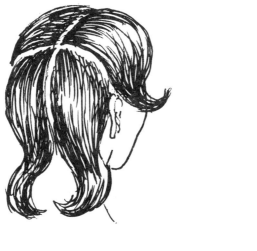

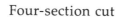

Four-section cut   Nape section separate

THINNING

You must first take into consideration the texture and quality of hair in the wig. Having done this, you can begin to thin. A very important step to successfully cutting a wig for a customer is the thinning. Wigs generally are made with more hair than necessary for style. This means that the excess hair will have to be thinned out until the proper amount of hair for the customer is reached. If your customer has fine thin hair she will not be able to carry as much hair as another with heavy hair.

Thinning with a Razor

When using a razor for thinning, the hair must be damp. Most of the bulk should be taken out very close to the cap so there will not be any short spurs sticking out when the wig is styled. Contrary to the customer's own hair, the wig hair will not continue to grow. Therefore, the hair cut close to the foundation will not grow to a length that will spur out beyond a style whether it be teased or soft and close to the cap. Hold strands of hair straight out between the middle and index fingers. Place the razor flat, not erect, with pressure on the back side of the razor, rather than on the edge. Use short, steady strokes toward the end of the hair.

Thinning with Thinning Shears

When using thinning shears, hair may be either damp or dry. When thinning close to the cap, hair should be dry. This will insure that all knots in hand-tied hair are tight and solid. You can see accurately how close you are cutting to a weft, and by feeling dry hair you can better judge how much bulk should be removed.

To thin, pick up a bunch of strands from one half to one inch thick. Holding the hair between your fingers, take thinning shears flat into the base of a hand tied wig (this also eliminates the bulk of extra knots on the cap). Move out from the base one or two inches, depending on the hair texture, and cut hair at a slight angle.

Wigs need more thinning or tapering around the face and temple area than at any other part of the wig. Strict attention should be paid to the bulk of hair that is to fit behind the ears. These areas are the very areas that are *never* thinned on a human head! Caution: The wefting on machine-made wigs cannot be cut into because this will disturb an entire row of hair. If the weft is cut into while thinning the hair, the entire row or weft of hair could unravel. If a very smooth, sleek hairstyle is your goal, do all necessary thinning at the base of the wig.

PROBLEM AREAS:

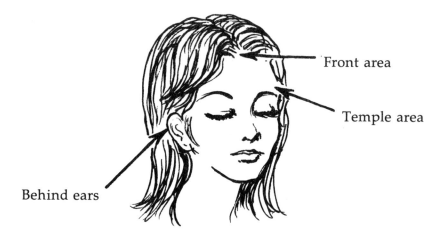

Front area

Temple area

Behind ears

In cutting wigs you must take many things into consideration. Some people like their wigs cut for one style only. Even if they want one type of cut, you must still section to thin, and readjust the sectioning for the haircut you and your customer decide on. Even if you have thinned at the base of the wig, you still will have to use the razor to texturize and taper the wig. The finer your customer's hair, the more you have to thin and taper. On most wigs you have more hair than you need to complete most hair styles. This applies not only to the one-style cut but also to all haircuts on wigs.

The cutting of hair pieces and falls is relatively simple after you decide on the style. They are cut mostly with scissors and without thinning. Falls may require some tapering at the bottom. Most of these pieces are sewn with some tapered lengths of hair in them. When in doubt, set the piece in the style and try it on the customer before you decide if it needs extra taper or not.

Cutting wigs, hairpieces, and falls is different from cutting a customer's hair. The basic rules must be learned, and then haircutting takes judgment and a lot of practice. You should not be afraid of making a mistake; you can often add hair if some portion of the wig is cut too short. The only thing you have to worry about is if the mistake is total.

By a total mistake we mean that you cut a wig, fall, or hairpiece much shorter than your customer and you have decided on for a style. Always remember, "more can be taken off," and often "enough cannot be put back on." It is a very good idea to cut a *guide* for a style or the length desired for a fall, on the customer's head. It is not a good idea to try to complete a cut on the head. Why? It is almost impossible to pin a wig, fall, or hairpiece on the head so that it will not give or slip to one side with pulling. Moving a piece so much as half an inch on either side of the head while cutting the hair could be that *total* mistake.

EXAMPLE 1:
Basic Haircut or Circle Cut

Part off four sections: Cut guide at center back, follow to left using ear lobe as guide on left. Continue back to right in same manner.

Guide completed, take down half of section 3.

Take section out to a 45° angle. Using neckline cut for guide, cut up, continue to left, and then complete lower half of section 4 the same way.

Cut bang area next. Judge lengths by the bridge of the nose.

Hold strand out from head; pick up guide from front hair, matching lengths by picking up strands from sections already cut. Match lengths with sides and back hair.

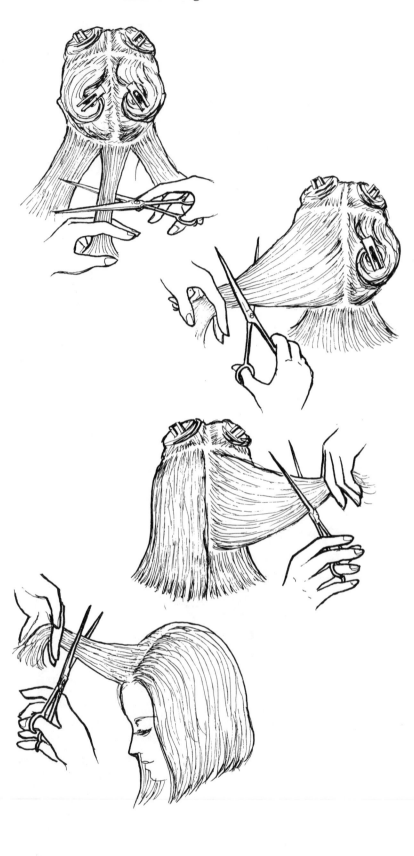

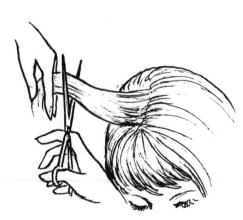

THE ADAPTABLE-STYLE CUT

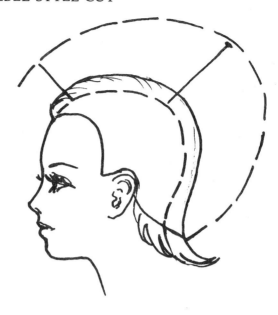

The front hair length will vary depending upon the style treatment around the face and the needs of the individual. The length of the hair at the crown will range from five to seven inches, and the length of the hair at the neckline will range from one to two and a half inches. Adapting the haircut professionally to the individual's requirements, both needs and preference, will result in a free and easy-to-care-for style.

EXAMPLE 2:
All-over Curl for Smooth and Short

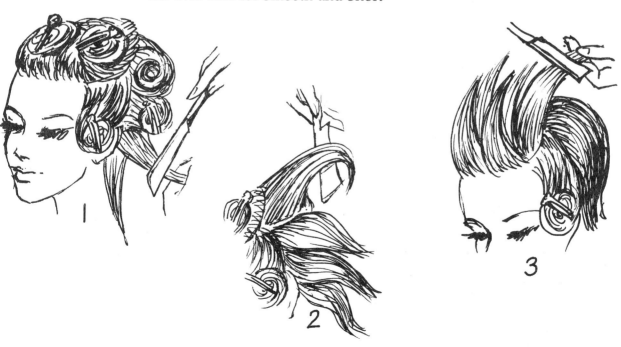

THE CUT.   Sketch 1, above, shows the arrangement of the hair sections into five areas which have to be taken into consideration in the cut. These areas are evenly pinned off, and then one after the other shortened by thinning. The bottom nape hair is thinned out so that it clings close and deep to the nape line.

In Sketch 2, section 2, over the nape, hair is thinned out in the last third of ½ inch sections. The hair graduates at the ends, remains full, and forms the transition to the nape line. In this way a well-formed profile of the back of the head is obtained. Section 3 on the top of the head shows the longest hair cover. Here the thinning out is performed in the last fourth of the hair from the bottom. The ends of the top hair may not be too long and too thin.

Sketch 3 shows the front hair (section 4) being picked up in individual ½ inch sections and in the direction of the coiffure, as in the other sections, shortened by thinning out. The hair is shortest in this section, except for that at the nape-line. The ½ inch sections are carefully tapered off; they, nevertheless, should appear full.

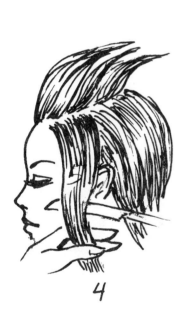

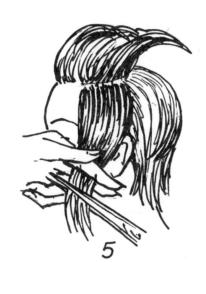

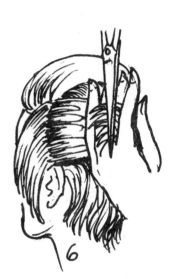

Neither of the side parts, sections 5, are thinned (see Sketch 4). The hair should remain full here and is brought to the necessary length with a few thinning-out cuts, about 1 to 1½ inches below the ear lobes. After the thinning-out cut of the side hair, the hair ends are checked for protruding thin tips by combing.

In Sketch 5, the cutter follows the blunt cut of the side-hair. The scissors are held in a vertical direction toward the nose. Sketch 6 shows the sections again being checked by combing; any protruding tips are then cut correctly in a blunt cut.

EXAMPLE 3:
Cheater cut

EXAMPLE 4:
Shag Cut

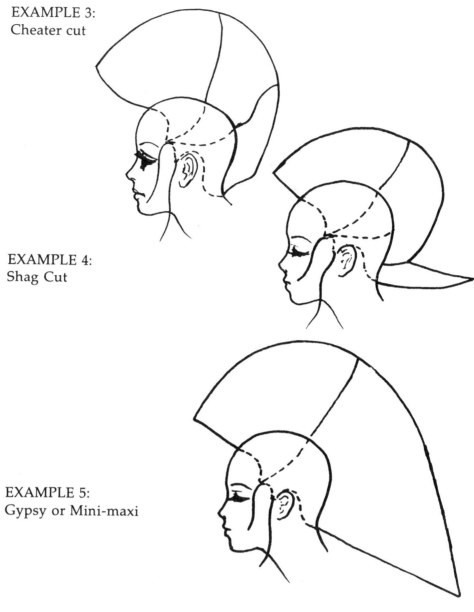

EXAMPLE 5:
Gypsy or Mini-maxi

EXAMPLE 6:
Cut for hair and hairpiece

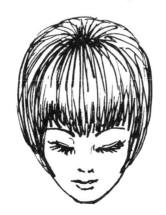

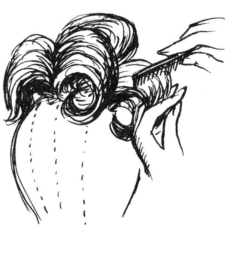

EXERCISE

1. Never cut a wig unless it is _____

2. Name the implements needed in hair cutting. A._____
   B. _____   C. _____   D. _____
   E. _____

3. Why should hair be sectioned before cutting? _____
   _____

4. What area is thinned on a wig that is never thinned on a human head?
   _____

5. List three problem areas in cutting a wig. A._____
   B. _____   C. _____

6. Why is it not advisable to cut a fall on a customer?_____
   _____

7. Where should most of the bulk be removed from a wig? _____
   _____

8. How is a razor held when thinning hair? _____
   _____

9. What is a good rule to remember in cutting a wig?_____
   _____

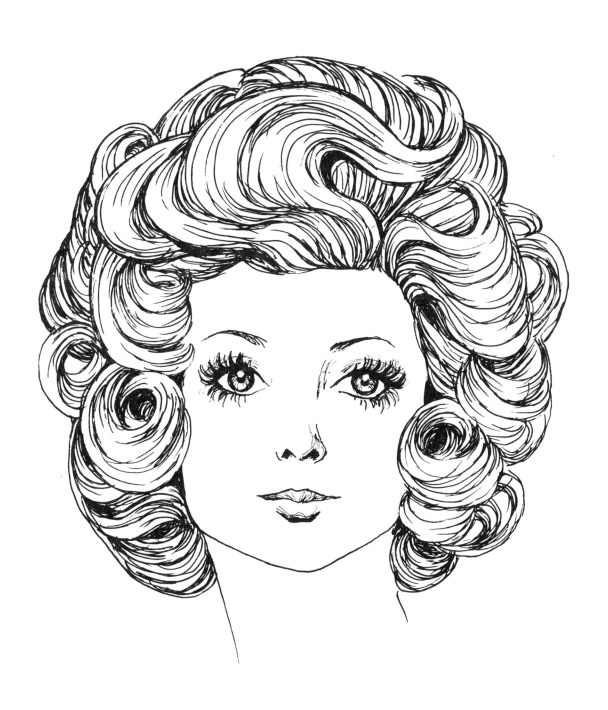

Chapter 6   # WIG
                                 # STYLING

The wigologist must have a good basic knowledge of hairstyles in order to keep his wig work as realistic as possible. The pin curl (also called flat curl or sculpture curl) is basic in the setting of wigs. It is usually used in areas where no height is needed. There are three basic parts of a pin curl and they should be studied in order to execute the proper placement and use of each part of the curl. These parts are: base, stem, and circle.

The base is the foundation of the curl, attached to the foundation of the wig cap. The stem consists of the hair between the foundation and the circle, and it gives the curl direction. The circle is the final part of the curl that forms a complete circle. The size of this circle determines the width of the wave and its strength. The ends should be inside the curl.

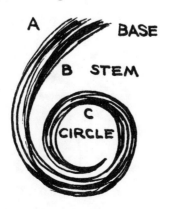

SAMPLE DRAWING OF A PIN CURL

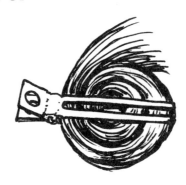

A curl and stem directed forward (called a C curl) will direct the hair toward the face; reversing this will direct the hair away from the face. Curls at the back of the head are directioned to the right or to the left.

PROCEDURE FOR PIN CURLS

The hair must be very wet with water or setting lotion and then combed smooth into the setting direction that forms line shapes. Curls are usually made by starting at the open end of a shaping. Shaping is the direction of hair used to create a line.

EXAMPLE:

section
sculptured
back for
shaping

open end
of shaping

strand wound into
forward C curl

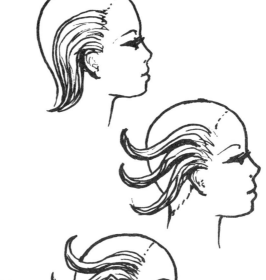

reverse
curls

completed
section of
C curls

stand up curls

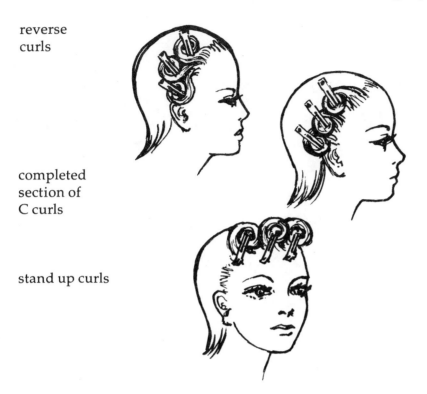

ROLLERS

Curls are also made with rollers; the size of the roller to be used is determined by the tightness or looseness of the curl desired. The larger the roller, the looser the curl will be.

EXAMPLES OF SIZES OF ROLLERS:

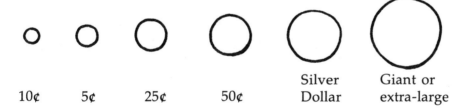

10¢   5¢   25¢   50¢   Silver   Giant or
                                          Dollar   extra-large

Smooth rollers with perforations are recommended for smoothest results and quicker drying time.

Tee pins are used to run through the perforations in the rollers, into the canvas block to secure the rollers. Note: Tee pins are preferred over clippies in order not to mark the hair.

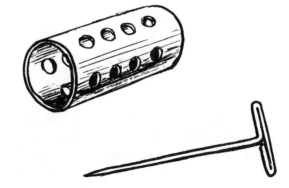

ROLLER TECHNIQUE
(Never lay down your comb.)

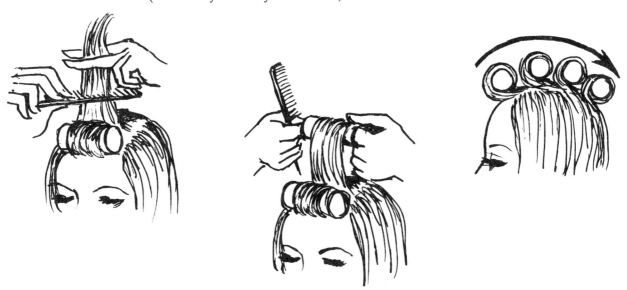

Wig styles should be carefully selected by you as a professional. This selection must not be left to your patron alone as she will need guidance in choosing a style for a full wig that is suitable for her. The lengths used in styling for each particular customer are most important. Do not let your customer talk you into doing something that you know is not going to be flattering to her because of her features, shape of face, length of forehead, neck or chin.

FACIAL STRUCTURES

There are seven facial patterns: oval, round, square, oblong, pear-shaped, heart-shaped, and diamond-shaped. For easier recognition these can be divided into four geometric designs.

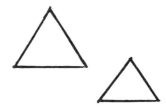

1. Triangle

A. PEAR-SHAPED.   This shape is characterized by a narrow forehead and a wide jaw line. Select styles that add width to the temple area and are close and short at the jaw line. If the fashions feature longer hair, use width at the temple, with hair pulled back from lower ear section and using nape area back interest or hair up.

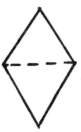

B. DIAMOND-SHAPED.   A narrow forehead, wide cheek bones, and narrow chin identify the diamond-shaped face. Choose styles that are full in the temple, close at the cheek (including hair brought onto the cheek) and that add width and softness at the jawline.

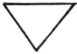

C. HEART-SHAPED.   The heart-shaped face has a wide forehead and a narrow chin. Use hair styles with low to left or right pivot or part carried to other side. Hair may also be dropped back onto the temples to make them appear more narrow and to add width at the jaw line.

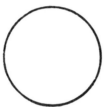

2. Circle

A round hairline and chinline characterize the circular face. Styles for this shape should be lifted in the center front, close-fitting along the temple, and flat on the cheeks or pulled behind the ears.

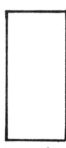

3. Rectangle

The rectangular face is long and narrow, often with a square jaw line. Select styles for it that stay fairly close to the top of the head and add fullness at the sides. Bangs, full or partial, are good; hair pulled back severely is not good. Jaw length hair is usually most flattering.

4. Square

The square face is characterized by a straight hairline across the forehead, wide temples with straight hairline, and a square jaw line. Choose styles that feature a lifted front, with hair dropped in close on temple, usually better on one side only. Hair should be soft and close, fitting out onto cheeks flat. An asymmetrical hair style (fullness on one side) is recommended for square and round faces.

Note: An oval face has generally been accepted as the perfect face, this shape being one and a half times longer than its width across the brow. The forehead is slightly wider than the chin. The most important factor in styles for this facial structure is the facial features. If any one feature should be minimized, brought out, or used as a focal point, a style should be created for this feature.

You are responsible for the styles your customer wears. Listen to her wants, likes, dislikes, and desires and combine them with your professional knowledge of styling to achieve the optimal solution.

STYLING PRODUCTS

In styling human hair goods, you have to know how to cut, set, and comb out, but most important to producing quality work, you must know the products to use on your hair goods to produce the results you desire.

SETTING LOTIONS.   A mild setting lotion can be used if you need it for extra body in the hair. *Rule:* If you use a good setting lotion you must dilute it with three times as much water as called for on the directions. If it says to use it straight, dilute it anyway. If used straight, the setting lotion will make the hair dry and brittle and very hard to comb, and you will have some breakage of the hair. To determine whether or not to use setting lotion depends on the style you are doing.

1. For a wig in simple style, water is best.
2. For a fall in simple style, flip or down, water is best.
3. On a hairpiece used as a filler, water is best.
4. For a hairpiece styled in long curls, setting lotion should be used.
5. On a hairpiece set into fancy curls, a setting lotion should be used.

Remember that when natural styles are wanted, water is the best and will also leave the hair with more luster.

HAIR SPRAY.   Affixative (spray net) must be water soluble and should have a fine mist and no lacquer. This type of high-quality spray can be used on both human hair and synthetic pieces. Caution: A lesser quality spray with lacquer will ruin the wig.

SETTING HUMAN HAIR GOODS

The hair should be soaking wet to obtain more strength to the set. Dry the hair on medium heat: this will take a little longer, but your results will be better and the curl will hold stronger. Try to set hair a day ahead of comb out.

QUICK, EMERGENCY SETTING.   There are three satisfactory methods to use for a quick, emergency set: (1) Dampen hair slightly and set. The curls will not be as strong as if they were set fully wet, but in an emergency you may have to do this. (2) Roll hair on heat rollers. (3) Use hot irons (curling irons); of the emergency measures, this is the best. (The use of curling irons will be explained in chapter 10.)

You are now ready to set a wig, but we have a few final cautions before you start. First, do not use rollers around the frame of the wig if you want or need to have the hair lay in close to the head. The shaded area is the caution area for rollers. Most of the time this area should be pincurled to have a closer fit of the hair.

EXAMPLE:

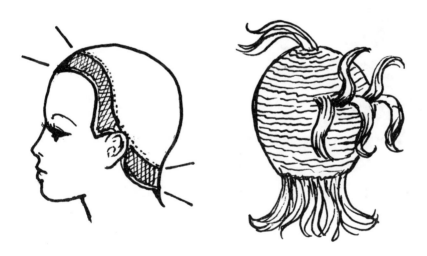

In setting a machine-made wig, be especially careful not to take roller sections directly down a row or weft. Instead, pick up hair on more than one row at a time in a zigzag fashion. If the hair is picked up on even rows and rolled onto the roller, the wefting is harder to conceal in the finished comb out because the rollers leave a wide indention at the base of the wig. Therefore, if the hair is picked up in zigzag sections from one weft to another, it has less tendency to gap into the original seams of the wig. This method holds true only on machine-made or semi-machine-made pieces.

BASIC SETS
AND SETTING PATTERNS

EXAMPLE 1

Half bang and no filler, uses customer's own hair on the left. C curl side on the left, soft C feather on right. Soft swirl back with fitted nape

Setting Pattern

Comb Out

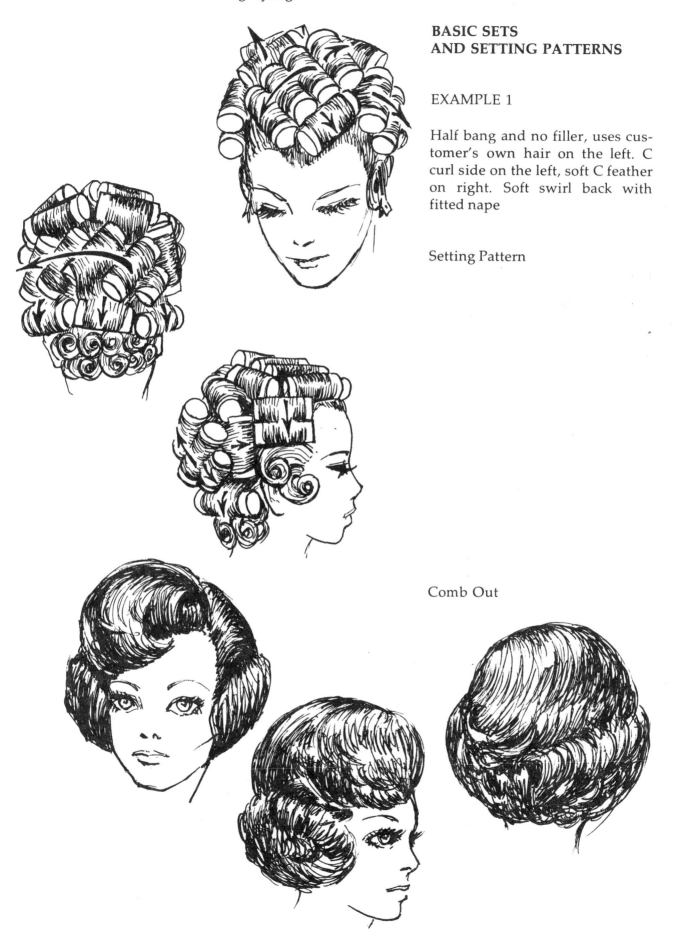

EXAMPLE 2

Soft, all-over curl look that completely covers hairline. Soft on
nape and fitted

Setting Pattern

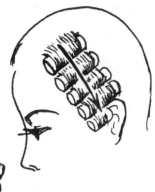

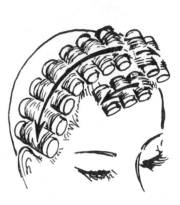

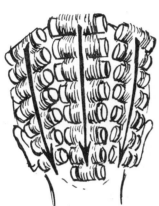

Comb Out

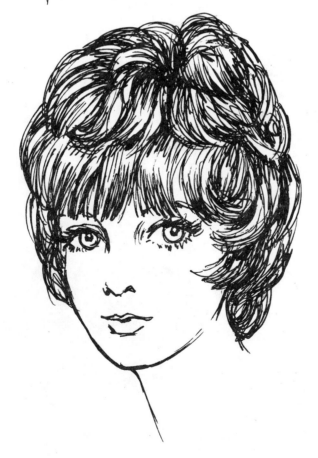

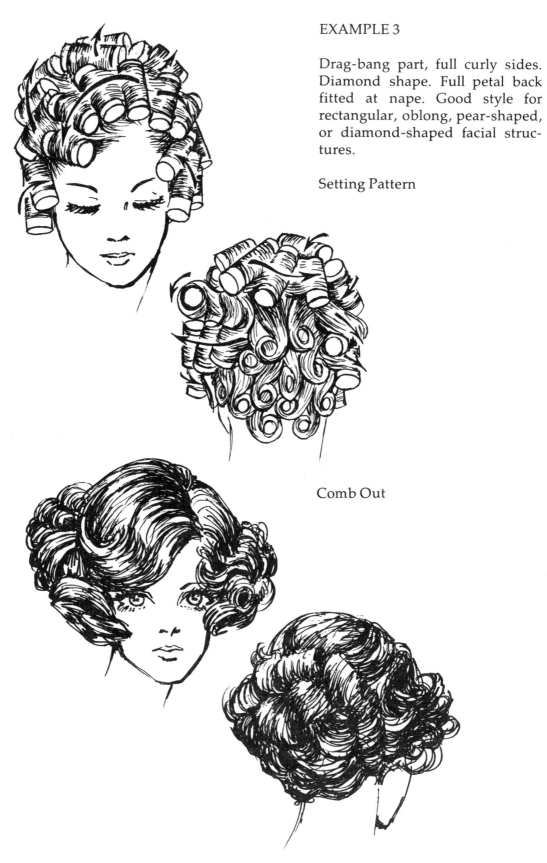

EXAMPLE 3

Drag-bang part, full curly sides. Diamond shape. Full petal back fitted at nape. Good style for rectangular, oblong, pear-shaped, or diamond-shaped facial structures.

Setting Pattern

Comb Out

EXAMPLE 4

Thin, fringy bangs, slightly curly
look; long guiche sides, and long
curly neck line.

Setting Pattern

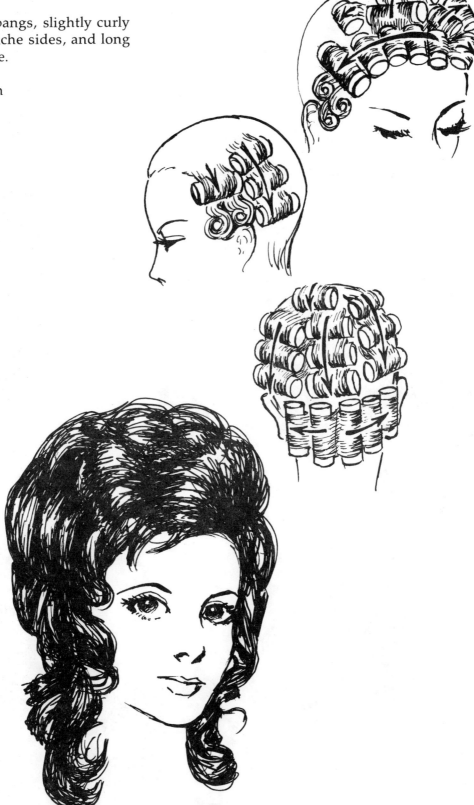

Comb Out

The hairstyles shown on this page are soft, classic styles that are relatively timeless.

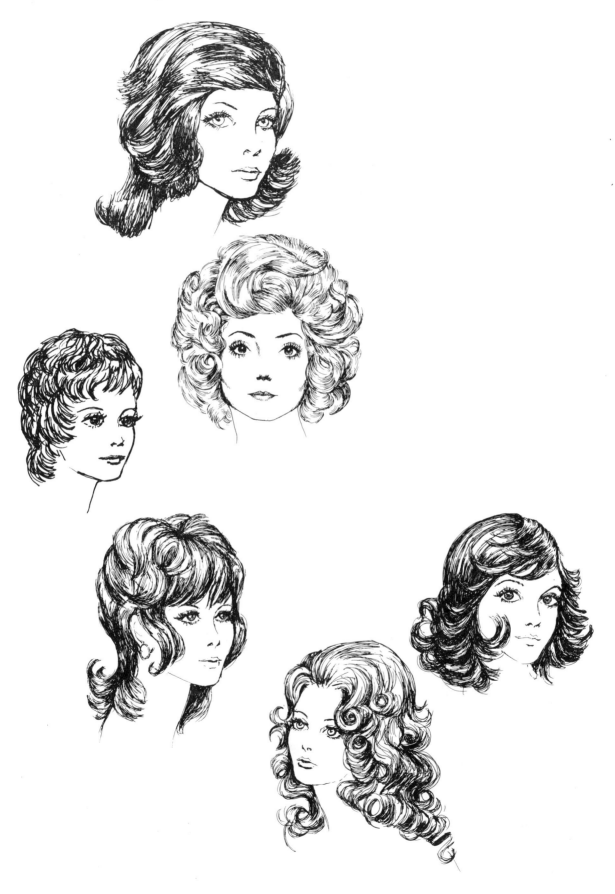

Hair Piece Styles

Flair Bun

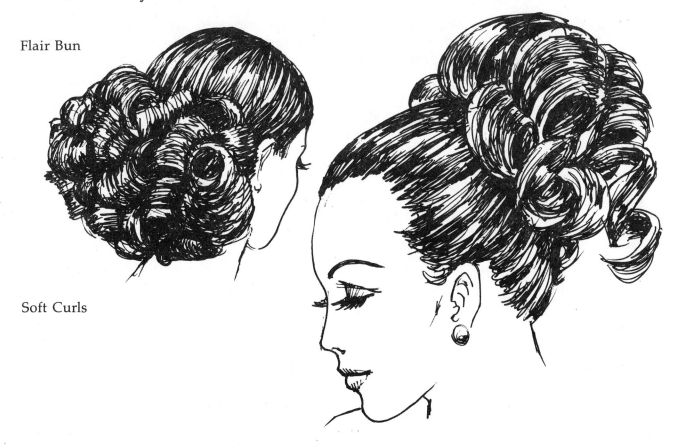

Soft Curls

Identification of Curls and Types of Comb Outs

Petal Curls	Flare Bun
Barrel Curls	Freedom Curls
Tucked Curls	Shirley Temple Curls
Swedish Braid	Spiral Curls
Ringlets	Basket Weave
Cascade Curls	Double Bun
Roll Curls	Triple Bun
Pinned in Curls	Psyche Knot
Grecian Curls	Spoolie Curls
Tossed Curl	Swedish Bun
Filler Petal	Curls and Braids
Filler	Bangs
Bun	Chignon
Figure Eight	Donut
Italian Top	Frou-Frou
Corkscrew	

SETTING HAIRPIECES, CASCADES, AND FALLS

When rolling a hairpiece, take into consideration the area on which it will be placed on the head, and roll with the thought in mind that this is only a partial hairstyle.

EXAMPLE:

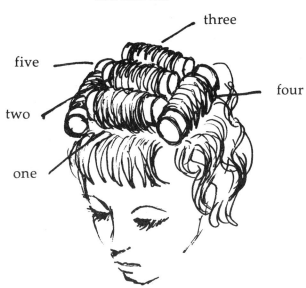

The top rollers only would be the hairpiece as it is going to be set in the customer's hairstyle and intermingled with her own hair when it is combed out.

If the hairpiece is to be used at the nape of the neck it may be placed on top of the canvas block for easier rolling, but you should remember where this piece is to be worn before the comb out is completed. The following examples are for normal use, but one should remember that there may be exceptions to all such rules. The nature of our business enables it to be run on an individual basis, and your professional knowledge and training will guide you in knowing when to follow the "rules" and when to make exceptions to them.

Simple, Basic Sets on Hairpieces

EXAMPLE:

Filler

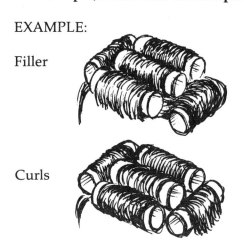

Curls

Five-roller set with hair going back on front rollers, down on sides.

Hair rolled forward on front roller, back on next two rollers, down on sides.

Caution: Do not place too much hair around rollers or use too large rollers. In order for the set to last, you need the curl obtained by using the proper number and size of rollers. Larger hairpieces will require more rollers, and this is preferable to trying to roll too much hair on each roller.

EXAMPLE:

Twelve-roller set with front hair all rolled back.

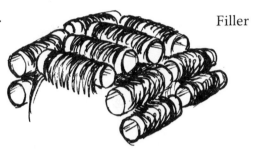

Filler

Twelve-roller set with front two rollers rolled forward.

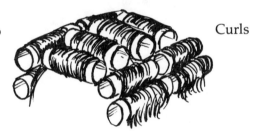

Curls

Swedish Braid

A Swedish braid is achieved by styling a hairpiece into a geometric pattern of curls without any loose ends. The setting pattern for the Swedish braid is like the setting pattern for curls, one roller forward and the rest back and down. For the comb out, brush the hairpiece and then tease. Take a one-inch section around the hairpiece and then clip the center hair together out of the way.

center
hair

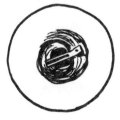

STEP 1.   Start the first curl in the front of the hairpiece. Brush the top hair smooth, and push the hair to the base with fingers, about one inch back. Pin parallel to edge. Roll the curl over toward you, gather the

ends of it together, looping under, and pin inside at the edge of the base. Take fingers and spread (like slinky) the center curl.

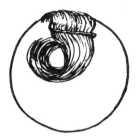

STEP 2.   Turn the hairpiece so you are parallel with the parting, pull number 2 hair section straight up with the top hair against the end of curl number 1. Brush top of hair smooth, push the hair flat to the base with finger about one inch back, and pin into the open end of curl number 1. This pin will be vertical to the end of curl number 1.

pin #2 inside curl #1

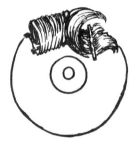 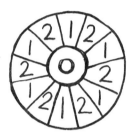

Roll the curl over in a barrel-like curl, grip hair ends together, and pin the inside of the curl at the edge of the base. Spread.

curl #1

pin curl #2 as #1

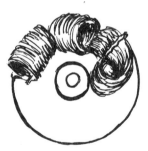

Complete this pattern all around the hairpiece, and you will have a woven look.

STEP 3.   Unclip the center hair. You will have enough hair for two or three curls. Smooth the top hair on either the two or three curls. Pin your base and make your barrel-roll curls in the center to fill in the finished style.

For a cascade styled in a Swedish braid, follow the same steps but complete the procedure twice because of the length of the base. First, divide the hairpiece into two sections, block off your center, and proceed with steps one, two, and three.

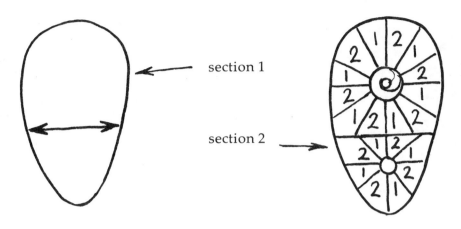

section 1

section 2

HAIRPIECE STYLES AND THEIR DIFFERENT PLACEMENT
ON THE HEAD

Two short small curly wiglets

Two short wiglets done
in bun styles

Small hairpiece done in bun

Small hairpiece
flare bun style

Small hairpiece done in tight
Psyche knot, or three barrel curls
turned into each other to form
cone shape.

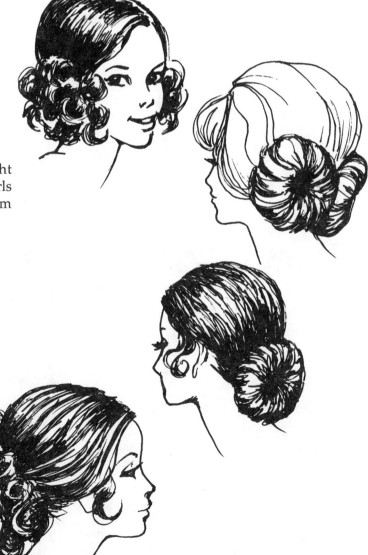

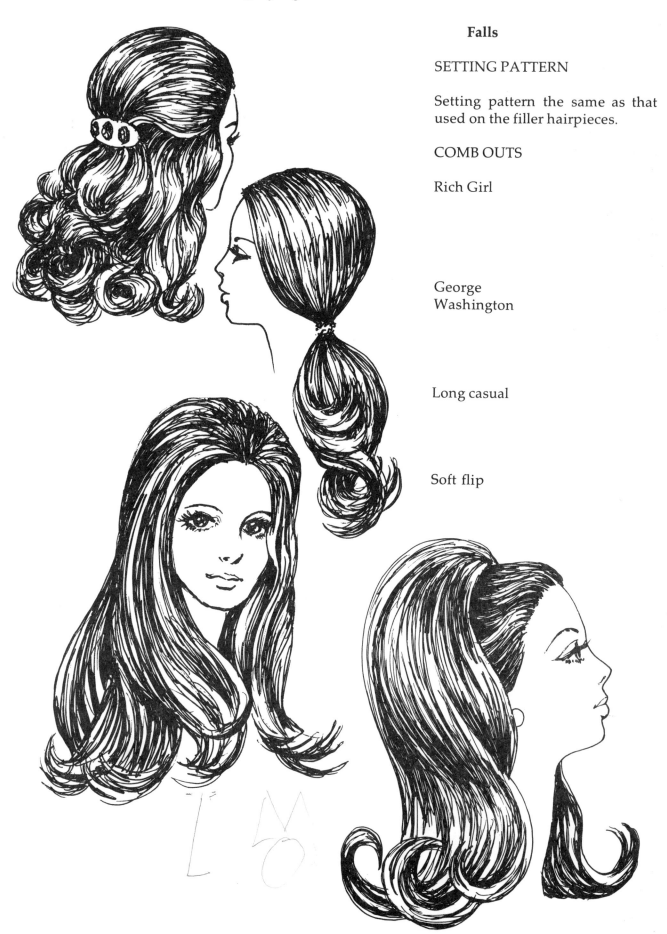

Falls

SETTING PATTERN

Setting pattern the same as that used on the filler hairpieces.

COMB OUTS

Rich Girl

George
Washington

Long casual

Soft flip

AFRO WIG

SWING STYLE

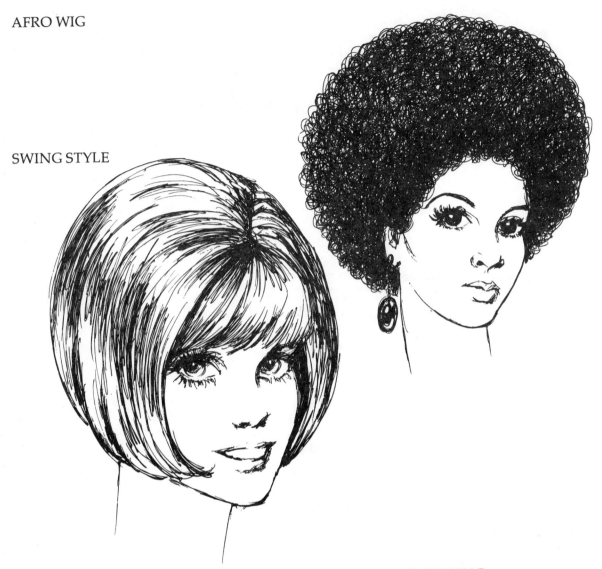

SYNTHETIC STYLING

Styling and caring for the synthetic wig has been a problem since the "synthetic rush" of 1968. Retail promoters educated the public to believe that all you must do to care for a synthetic wig is to wash it in a cold-water fabric cleaner, dry, shake out, and the style would return to the wig. This is far from the truth, and you will find that servicing synthetic wigs can be as tricky and as much a professional problem as servicing human-hair wigs.

First, synthetics should never be washed in anything other than a mild wig shampoo. Cleaning a synthetic in a liquid wig cleaner solution will destroy all the elastic in the cap. Products perfected for cold-water cleaning have a tendency to leave a build up on the fiber after a series of cleanings. Tepid water should be used, since the fiber and cap can be damaged by hot water. Never comb a synthetic wig when it is wet; some of the fibers may stretch if you do so, and some of the curl will be taken out.

When cutting a synthetic, never use a razor. Synthetic fiber is solid, and not having a cuticle like human hair, it will not react like hair to a razor cut. Thinning shears or tapering shears with a fine tooth will give you more success in cutting; they will minimize the possibility of a total blunt or choppy cut. An experienced slither cut with regular shears is very good. For more information, refer back to the haircutting chapter.

Teasing or backcombing of synthetic fibers is very different from human-hair teasing. It should be concentrated solely at the base of the fiber in order not to damage the fiber that should remain smooth at the surface of the wig. If this is not done, the wig will frizz or become fuzzy-looking all over.

Some stretch wigs will have to be sized just as your human-hair caps are sized. This should be done before any additional cutting is done to the wig. Refer back to the chapter on sizing and blocking.

Styles should be carefully selected since all synthetics are pre-cut into definite styles at the factory. Even though you may select a short tapered cut with longer hair lengths at the neckline for your customer, this wig has the potential to be combed out in many different styles. A professional wig stylist might comb the cut in a bubble or a half-bang filler with a wing side. The synthetic really never needs setting, and the possible style variations are limited only by the ability of the comb-out artist.

If it is your job to sell a synthetic wig and then service it, be sure you select one of the finest quality. In making this selection, consider not only the quality of the fiber itself but also the climatic conditions in which you live. Some fibers do better than others in hot climates, and some are better in extreme cold. In general, the lifetime of a synthetic (worn often) is much shorter than that of human hair.

WIG DRYERS

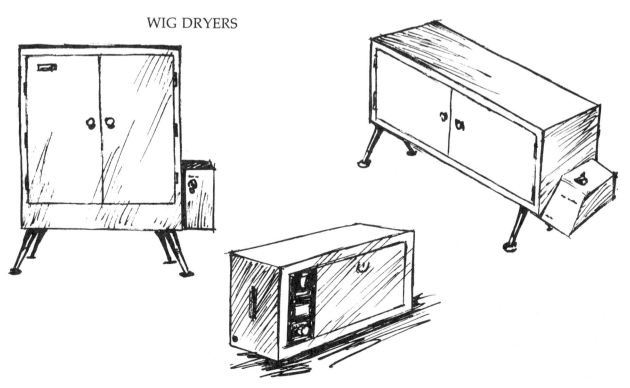

DRYING

Drying time for wigs is an important factor in the preservation of processed hair. Lengthy drying time is required, and blond pieces especially should never be placed in extreme heat. Better sets are realized from a slower drying process. Use only medium heat for drying of all pieces.

Regular wig dryers are the most successful in wig salons because not only do they provide a regulated heat, but also they can dry many pieces at one time.

"PUT ON'S"

In the wig business the "put on" is a very familiar term. Once a wig or hairpiece has been completely styled, the wigologist puts this piece on the customer and balances it to the customer's likes and facial features.

The hairpiece has been styled on a canvas block. The canvas block, even though the best method in styling hairgoods, has its disadvantages because it doesn't show you the size or the face shape of the customer. The piece may be beautiful and perfect on the block and the style may fit the style description exactly, but the hairpiece may not look good on the customer for whom it has been designed. Thus, it is essential that the wigologist take the hairpiece, place it on the customer's head, and make any necessary adjustments. The "put on," then, not only will satisfy the customer, but the wigologist can be sure that the customer likes the work and that she will continue to be a customer.

HOW TO PUT ON A WIG

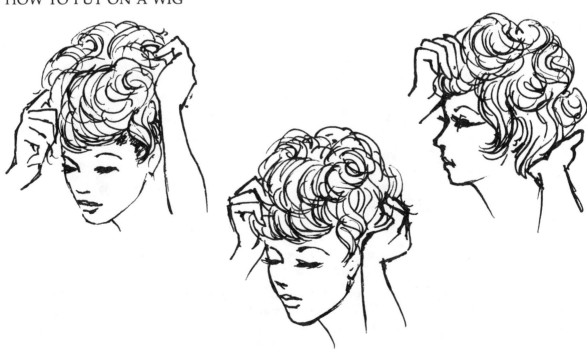

How to Place a Hairpiece

If the hairpiece is done in curls you must decide, along with your customer, where the piece looks best on her head. You tease and pin up the customer's own hair in a position where the hairpiece will cover the pins, and then place it on her head. When the style is a filler you must fit it into her hair style. The different placement of the piece can produce many style looks.

EXAMPLES:

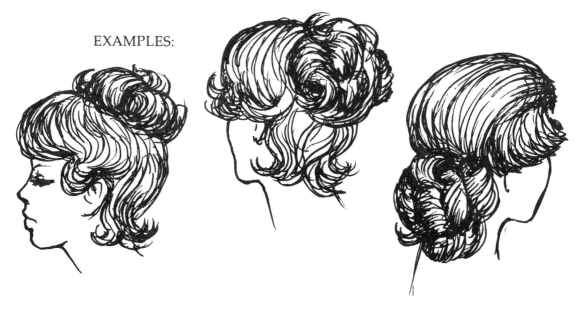

All of the styles above use the same curl style, and a great many of your customers would want this many style changes with the same piece. Falls are placed on the head like a hairpiece. Again, consider the style of the fall, arrange the customer's hair accordingly, and place your piece.

EXAMPLES:

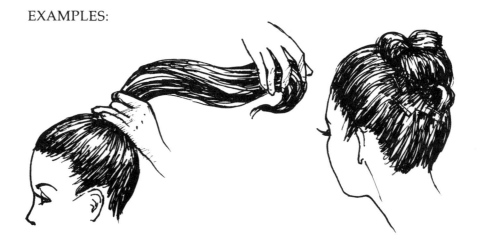

In salon custom-styling of hairgoods, the "put on" is one of the most important contacts you have with your customer. This is where you please her with your work, sell to her, and build a lasting relationship. Even though you may be very busy with other things, the "put on" is well worth the effort. Not every customer will want to "put on" each time, but leave time available if she desires this service. You will find that the customer with whom "put on" contact is made is a much better salon customer than one who only picks up her pieces. The one who picks up may be unhappy with the work, not because it was not done right, but because she doesn't know what to do with it. How will you ever know what your customer feels about your work, if you do not do the "put on"?

EXERCISE

1. Name the 3 parts of a pin curl. A. _____ B. _____
   C. _____

2. What does the size of the circle of a pin curl determine? _____
   _____

3. What is a C curl? _____

4. What is a shaping? _____

5. Give four geometric facial shapes. A. _____
   B. _____ C. _____ D. _____

6. Can setting lotions be used on wigs? _____

7. Is lacquer ever used on wigs? Explain. _____
   _____

8. Are wigs placed in hot dryers? Why? _____
   _____

9. Name 3 ways to set for emergency sets. A. _____
   B. _____ C. _____

10. What should be different in the setting of hand-tied wigs and machine-made wigs? _____
    _____

11. What is a Swedish braid? _____
    _____

12. Why are tee pins recommended for attaching rollers instead of clippies? _____

13. Why should hair be soaking wet when set? _____
    _____

14. Where is a caution area on a wig about to be set? _____
    _____

15. Are synthetic wigs rolled? _____

16. Will a synthetic wig last as long as a human-hair wig? _____

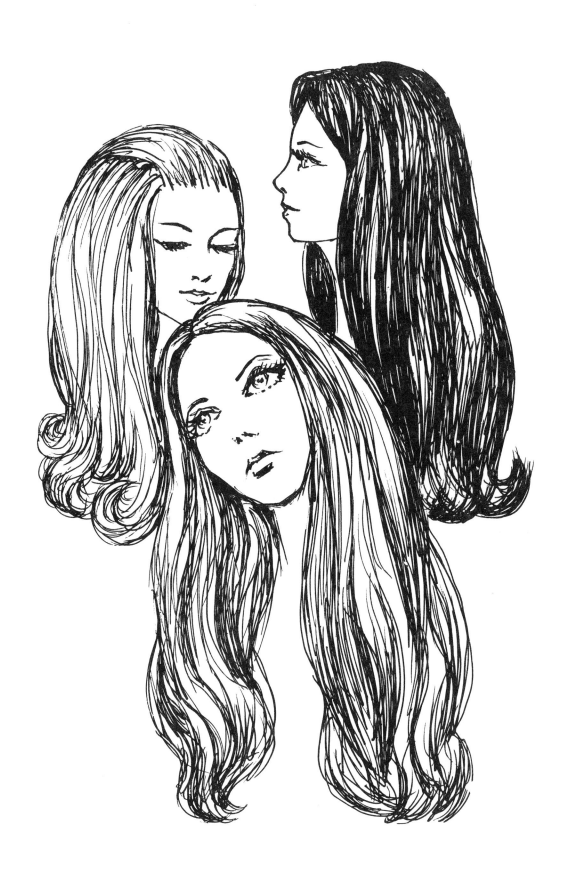

Chapter 7

WIG COLORING

WIG COLORS

Wig colors are referred to by a number. These numbers have been reduced to one international color ring, used by all manufacturers, and without a knowledge of these colors and their descriptions, it would be very difficult to function well in selecting colors and matching these colors with your customer's hair. This color ring is named the J and L color ring, and is believed to have been originated by two Frenchmen named Jacques and Lameaux in the nineteenth century. It is used for all types of hair from European to Oriental and also by the larger manufacturers of synthetics. There are approximately 70 colors listed on the ring at this time and it will probably be revised occasionally to eliminate colors not in demand or to add new colors that, with a season, have become widely used and standardized.

Listed here are the J and L color numbers with a description of color shade:

1. Jet Black
1b. Off-black
2. Darkest brown
3. Very dark brown

4. Dark brown
5. Medium dark brown
6. Chestnut
7. Medium brown

8. Brown
9. Walnut
10. Medium walnut
11. Light walnut
BR Bright red
12. Extra-light walnut
13. Dark ash brown
14. Medium ash brown
15. Light ash brown
16. Honey blonde
17. Darkest ash brown
18. Ash brown
19. Dark ash blonde
20. Medium ash blonde
21. Beige blonde
22. Light beige blonde
23. Swedish blonde
24. Golden blonde
25. Wheat blonde
26. Light dirty blonde
27. Sun bronze
28. Dark sun bronze
29. Light bronze
30. Copper
31. Light copper
32. Auburn
33. Dark auburn
34. Off-black/gray mix
35. Darkest brown/gray mix
36. Dark brown/gray mix
37. Chestnut/gray mix
38. Light chestnut/gray mix

39. Light off-black/gray mix
40. Brown/gray mix
41. Light brown/gray mix
42. Dark chestnut/gray mix
43. Medium chestnut/gray mix
44. Salt and pepper
45. Light salt and pepper
46. Walnut/gray mix
47. Medium walnut/gray mix
48. Light walnut/gray mix
49. Medium light walnut/gray mix
50. Light ash blonde/gray mix
51. Silver gray mix
52. Silver ash/gray mix
53. Ash/gray mix
54. Ash blonde/gray mix
55. Beige blonde/gray mix
56. Light silver/gray mix
57. Light beige blonde/gray mix
58. Silver blonde/gray mix
59. Platinum blonde/gray mix
60. White silver
101. Silver beige
102. Golden beige
103. Pink beige
104. Ash beige
105. Medium ash beige
106. Platinum beige
107. Silver ash

WIG COLOR FROM THE BEGINNING

Before attempting to color any processed hair, one should have an understanding of what has already been done to this hair. Some hair cannot and will not accept any additional color. Some hair cannot and will not go to a lighter shade. There are many different factory processes; the one described below is a typical method.

The hair is sorted as to quality and length, and washed in cool water. It is then placed in a bleaching solution known as a German white bleach, which is ten times as strong as your powder bleach. The hair is bleached as light as it will go and still remain strong. The bleached hair is then washed again, dried, and sorted according to the color or bleaching stage it has reached. The lightest of these is a corn-yellow called #613. The loose hair is then taken in bunches, and the root end is dipped into wax about six inches up the shaft. This is allowed to solidify and is then lowered on large wire strainers into the desired color, these colors being only red, yellow, brown, black, and white. The wax makes the root end float, and the hair sinks straight into the color. The dyes used are crystal, being similar to fabric dyes, and some of these have a metallic base. No color shades are determined, until after the hair is removed from the dye and dried. The hair is then matched and tagged by color number of the J and L color ring. It is then ready to be shipped to different wig manufacturers who do the sewing or hand-tying to the caps. The metallic-base dyes are the biggest problem in re-coloring any processed hair. The color change can only be made if you understand how to remove the present dye and apply the new.

The first and most important rule in using any method of coloring is to know your product; determine whether it is human hair or synthetic, machine-made or hand-tied. Human hair will accept color rinses, tints, and sometimes hair lighteners. Synthetic hair will sometimes accept a vegetable rinse. No tint or bleach should be used on synthetics at this time. Machine-made pieces are easier to color because of the construction of the piece. The hair cannot back up through the cap, but it can tangle or mat badly through the foamy action of most tints. Be very careful that a hand-tied wig is blocked tightly before applying any color or tint. Remove all color with dry-cleaning solution before rinsing with water in order to keep the knots from becoming loose or open. Always make a timed test strand before applying color or tint to *any* wig or hairpiece. The color time on processed hair is usually about one-half of regular color time. Color will appear lighter when wet and dry to a darker shade.

RINSES

Vegetable rinses are easily applied. They need no peroxide, and will stay on the hair only until it is re-wet or cleaned. Basically, they are used for the following reasons:

1. To give more depth to a color.
2. To drab out gold in some blonde shades.
3. To eliminate the yellow in gray or salt-and-pepper hair.
4. To temporarily add color to faded hair or sun-streaked hair.

Application

After you have cleaned, conditioned, and blocked your wig, hairpiece, or fall, the hair should be wet, combed smooth, towel blotted, and the rinse applied full strength. Start at the nape area, combing rinse through each layer of hair as it is laid down. Continue working each layer completely around to the side of the wig.

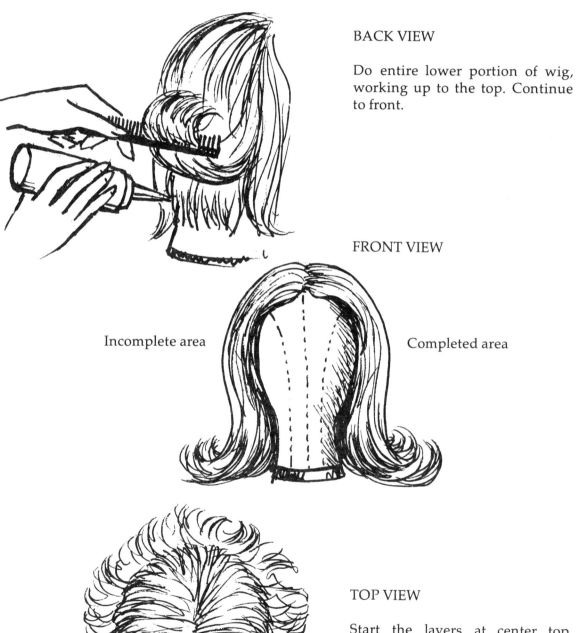

BACK VIEW

Do entire lower portion of wig, working up to the top. Continue to front.

FRONT VIEW

Incomplete area   Completed area

TOP VIEW

Start the layers at center top crown, combing layers down onto each other until front layer is combed last. Set in usual manner, dry, and comb out.

A rinse is a coating type of color and often leaves the hair dull-looking. This fact should be taken into consideration and explained to your customer. She then will have a better understanding of what the end product will be and will not be likely to be disappointed that it was not as she had imagined.

SEMI-PERMANENT COLOR

Determine whether the wig is human hair or synthetic. Semi-permanent colors are not recommended for any synthetic at this time. The most successful and widest used of all hair coloring on wigs and hairpieces, is the semi-permanent color, sometimes referred to as six-week colors. These colors do not require peroxide. The advantages of semi-permanent colors are that they

1. are easier to apply;
2. will often last as long as a permanent color;
3. leave the hair in a better condition than do permanent colors;
4. will not rub off on clothing;
5. are easier to correct if any mistakes occur.

Application

All machine-made pieces may be colored off the block. You will need the following equipment: a glass or porcelain bowl, a wide-tooth comb, and the color. First, remove all teasing, tangles, and snarls. Clean the wig and comb smooth. Place four ounces of hot water for smaller pieces, eight ounces of hot water for larger pieces in the bowl. Mix one or two ounces of color depending on the depth of color needed (test by eye to determine). Immerse entire wig or piece into bowl and be certain that all hair is saturated. Leave the hair immersed for ten minutes. At the end of this interval, remove the piece and rinse thoroughly with cool water. This helps set your color. If additional conditioner is needed, apply it now. Block the wig or hairpiece, set it in the usual manner, dry, and comb out.

Note: Remember when checking colors on any processed hair (all wig and hairpiece hair has been processed) that the color will appear *lighter* when wet and will dry to a darker shade. The only exception to this is in the case of a vegetable color rinse.

PERMANENT COLOR

Permanent colors are aniline-derivative tints, also called organic-penetrating tints.

Application

Wrap block in plastic to protect it. Place the wig or hairpiece on the block, using tee pins to secure it. Make sure all snarls, tangles, and teasing have been removed from the hair. Dampen hair slightly and towel blot. Section the hair into four parts. Begin applying the color to the nape

Back section

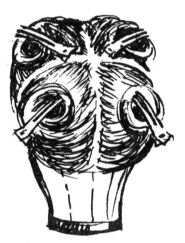

area first, working up to the center crown. Next, do the side area from the crown down to the ear. Repeat this on the second side, and then work front to the bang area. Finally, run the color around the edge of the entire wig. Comb the color evenly through the hair, and set a timer. All aniline-derivative tints should be used per the manufacturer's instructions for mixing, but timing should be determined by a test strand only. We suggest a fifteen minute color check. Remember that the hair will appear lighter when wet and will dry to a darker or deeper tone.

Color may be removed from all machine-made hairpieces with a small amount of mild shampoo. Take care to rub shampoo in a downward direction and rinse with a lot of tepid water. Towel blot, comb hair smooth, remove from block, and check that all color has been removed from around the cap edge and the interior of the cap. Color left inside the wig or weft will cause quick deterioration of the cap if the wig is set and dried without removing this color.

Hand-tied wigs may be rinsed thoroughly with tepid water. Towel blot and then follow with a complete cleaning with liquid dry-cleaning solution. The inside of the cap should be checked after combing the hair smooth. Change the covering on the block, re-block, condition if necessary, and set as usual.

Note: All human-hair pieces will retain their luster and beauty for a much longer period if they are not dried at extreme hot temperatures.

COLOR REMOVAL ON WIGS

First, determine whether the product is human hair, hand-tied, or machine-made. Synthetics cannot be lightened at this time. Color removal on certain wigs does become necessary at times. The first point that should be reviewed is the fact that some wig dyes do have a metallic base. Second, all wigs (unless labeled virgin hair) have previously been bleached and then colored. Blonde shades are usually more easily stripped of some color. There are several methods of color removal.

METHOD 1.   Some color can be removed from all shades with a stripping or detergent shampoo. This should be done carefully and tested first on a small section to see the reaction of the hair. Check for snarling or excessive tangling of the hair. This can be done by putting a small amount of shampoo on a section of hair and rubbing slightly with the fingers. If the hair continues to back up and mat in tight knots, it is wiser to tell your customer that color removal on her hair piece is not safe. If at this point you feel you will be able to control the hair, make sure it is free of all teasing and tangles before proceeding. Immerse the hair in warm water with fingers underneath the hair and securely holding the base on *both* sides. Run fingers from base out to ends of hair and continue checking for tangling. Again gently run fingers from base to hair ends working shampoo all along the shaft. This soaking should continue for three to five minutes. Again holding the hairpiece at the base with your fingers through the hair from the underneath side, take the spray and run water *through* the base of the hair so that the hair is streaming straight out from the base. Rinse thoroughly. Dry hair to see exactly what shade and tone have been arrived at before applying additional color. The hair may be re-dampened before applying new color, as color does take faster on processed hair. Always make a timed test strand before applying to the full piece. This method is used for all pieces needing a slight change of color or about two shades in different color tone.

All lighter blondes need fillers and conditioners. All coloring should be concluded with an acid rinse to reharden the hair and prevent tangling before setting. A good acid rinse may be made by combining 1 ounce vinegar to 8 ounces of water.

METHOD 2.   Use a professional product called a stripper. Remember here that all hand-tied pieces must be blocked tightly on a canvas block and hair kept smooth to prevent the hair from backing through cap, or matting, or the knots becoming loose. The stripper is applied directly onto wet hair and worked into the hair as you would a shampoo. It remains on 15 to 20 minutes. Rinse it out and dry a section to determine if the hair has lightened sufficiently to receive new color or toner. Remember: The hair will have a lighter appearance when wet than when dry.

METHOD 3.   If more color removal is necessary on brown, red, or black colors, combine two parts 20 volume hydrogen peroxide with one part stripper, and apply to smooth, dampened hair. Work through the hair from the base out to the ends of the hair and leave on 20 to 25 minutes, checking the processing at 10-minute intervals. Make sure the hair is not in a draft. Wrap it loosely in plastic to speed the color removal action. Rinse thoroughly with tepid water, checking the elasticity of the hair, and dry it thoroughly before applying filler, conditioner, or color.

METHOD 4.   Metallic dye solvents are available and should be used only according to the manufacturer's instructions. These dye solvents will remove all metallic dye substances from the hair and will take it back to the dark yellow stage (sometimes leaving only a pink stain), but should be used with caution. Be sure to do a time test strand before determining the condition the hair will be in at its final stage. These solvents are harsh and should be used with utmost care and consideration of your customer's hair piece. Conditioning will be necessary. After color removal, dry the hair (do not use hot dryers) and check it before adding new color. Again perform a strand test.

METHOD 5.   Hair bleaches and lighteners that are mixed with hydrogen peroxide may be used if tested first. This will give a more lightening effect to most hair. Apply as directed by the manufacturer and condition and dry before applying analine-derivative color or semipermanent color. Make sure that all lightener is cleaned completely from the cap or weft as this could cause deterioration of the cap.

METHOD 6.   The sixth method of color removal is powder bleaching. This is *not* recommended for wigs. If light frosting or streaking is desired, it is safer to sew the lighter hair in blocks or strips into wig than to use a powder bleach. This can be done with wefts of hair in the right shade.

Frosting

Wigs or hairpieces may be pulled through the cap and frosted as any human head of hair. Block the piece securely on the canvas block. Brush all hair back smooth from front of the cap, cover with a plastic cap and then with a frosting cap. Starting at front hairline, pull strands of hair through cap with a crochet needle working back to the crown, down the temple area to the ear, and doing the back section last. Liquid hair lightener may be used, but do not use powder bleach. Do test a strand to determine timing before you apply lightener. When the color is removed, wash off *without removing cap*. Towel blot, and check the elasticity and strength of the hair. Proceed with toner on damp hair, and wash off with *cool* water. Remove the cap, and smooth out the hair. Again rinse *thoroughly* with cool water. Check inner cap, re-block, set, and dry in a cool dryer.

1. What is the international color ring that is used by all the major wig manufacturers? _____

2. What is the meaning of the term *processed hair?* _____
   _____

3. What is a vegetable rinse? _____

4. Define semi-permanent color. _____

5. Can synthetic wigs take semi-permanent color?_____

6. Why is a semi-permanent color rinsed with cool water? _____
   _____

7. Are all permanent colors mixed with peroxide? _____

8. What is an aniline-derivative color? _____

9. Should hand-tied pieces be blocked before coloring? _____

10. Will color appear lighter or darker when wet? _____
    _____

11. To what area do you begin applying color to first? _____

12. State briefly three methods of color removal. A. _____
    B. _____ C. _____

13. Can metallic dyes be removed? _____

14. Is it safe to use powder bleach on wigs? _____

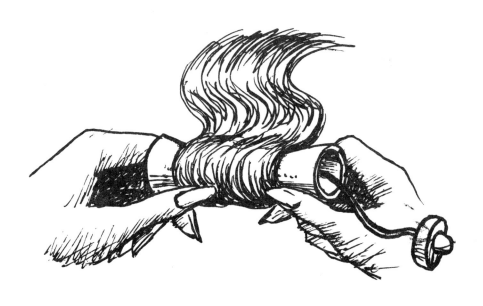

Chapter 8 PERMANENT WAVING

In most cases, human hair is treated to give it a semi-permanent wave before it is made into the finished hairpiece. This is usually done by wrapping the hair around a rod while heat and a waving solution are applied. Most human-hair wigs and hairpieces can be satisfactorily permanent-waved using the standard cold waving process. Synthetic hair, however, cannot be cold waved.

COLD WAVING

Cold waving is a method of permanent waving hair that uses chemical waving solutions and neutralizer or hardening solutions. No heat is required or desired. Cold wave solutions of various brand names are available. With a few special exceptions, they are made of basically the same chemicals. Some have buffering agents added to soften the harshness of the waving process and are available in various solution strengths. For purposes of permanent waving wigs and hairpieces, you should usually choose the solution strength for bleached and porous or damaged hair.

TEST CURLS. Before attempting to permanent wave a wig or hairpiece, the entire cold wave process should be completed on one or two test curls in order to determine:

1. The porosity of the hair.
2. The actual damage done by the original bleaching in the factory processing of the hair.
3. The amount of discoloration of the hair, if any, caused by the presence of metallic dyes.
4. The amount of time required to obtain the proper amount of curl.
5. The advisability of applying the permanent wave to the tested wig or hairpiece.

If the test curls indicate that a cold wave can be applied to the tested wig or hairpiece with satisfactory results, then proceed with the cold wave. If the test curls show damage or discoloration, DO NOT proceed.

EXAMPLE:

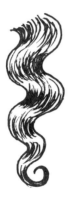 Good results

 Porous frizzy ends, over-processed; do not proceed.

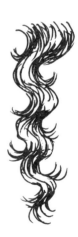 Breakage; do not proceed

PERMANENT WAVE PROCEDURE

The first step in permanent waving is to make certain that the hairpiece has a good, even haircut. The ends should be even in order to wrap the hair evenly and obtain the desired curl without causing dry, unruly ends.

Sectioning for Cold Waving

Block the wig properly, wet it thoroughly, and towel dry. Then part the hair into sections as illustrated.

EXAMPLE:

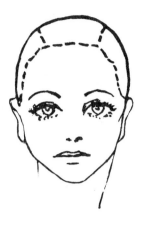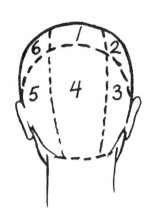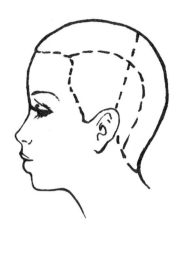

Proper Curler Selection and Placement

The size of the tightness of the wave is determined by the size of the curler used. The larger the diameter of the curler, the larger or looser the wave. The smaller the curler, the tighter the wave pattern will be. Therefore, choose your curlers carefully. Generally you should use larger diameter curlers at the top and crown sections, graduating them in size to smaller curlers at the lower temple and nape areas.

EXAMPLE:

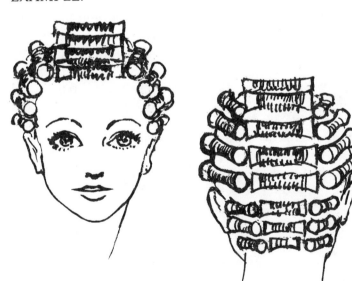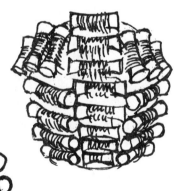

Wigs are parted off into six sections: one top; two front sides; one center back; two back sides. Wiglets and other hairpieces should be parted in the desired sections in a uniform manner.

Wrapping the Hair onto the Curler and
Applying the Curling Solution

Starting, preferably in the back center sections, pick out lateral sections about one half inch wide and two inches across. Comb through to smooth the strand and bring the ends to a point.

EXAMPLE:

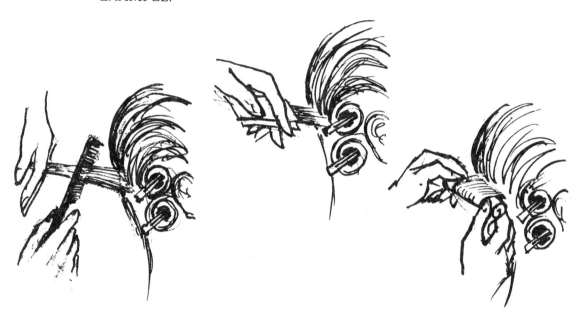

Apply one endpaper to the underside of the strand and one to the top-side. With your forefinger on top and your index finger under, slide the papers down the strand until the ends of the paper extend at least one quarter to one half inch past the end of the strand. Use your thumb and index finger of the other hand to start to roll the end of the paper and hair strand around the curler. Continue to roll the curler toward the block, using no tension at all, because this hair will stretch even more when you add the waving solution, possibly causing additional breakage. Be careful, too, to choose the proper diameter of curler for each section being rolled, and to divide each section of hair to be rolled into the proper thickness for the roller selected. Generally, the basic permanent wave is achieved by sectioning the hair into strands the same thickness as the curler. As you complete the wrapping of the hair, pour your waving solution into a plastic squeeze bottle and apply it to each wrapped curl evenly.

Testing for Wave Pattern and Firmness

Wigs will usually process very, very quickly. Test your curls for the proper wave pattern using the following method:

TESTING THE CURLS

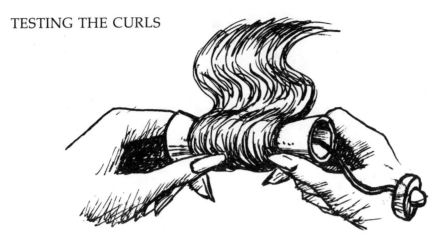

1. Loosen the fastener.
2. Unwind the curler several turns.
3. With the thumb, hold the hair on the curler and push toward the base of the strand.
4. Observe the amount of curl already formed; rewind the curl.

As the processing continues the wave formation will become stronger until it forms a strong letter "S". Further processing will cause the wave pattern to buckle which indicates the beginning of the hair being over-processed and permanently damaged.

Rinsing and Blotting the Curls

When the desired "S" pattern is reached, the curlers should be rinsed thoroughly with tepid water for several minutes, using a small amount of water pressure. This step will stop the waving process. Blot each curler with a towel by laying a dry towel over the block, and with your fingers, blot each curl to remove as much water as possible. *This process is very important.* Blot again if necessary.

Pour your neutralizer solution into a plastic squeeze bottle and apply it to each curl, first to the inside of the curler through the hole in the fastener and then to the outside. Apply the solution generously, making certain every curl is saturated. Allow the recommended time for the neutralizer to remain on the curl. You cannot overneutralize, so it is better to be a little generous with the time allowed.

Removing Neutralizer and Curlers

When the neutralizing time has elapsed, rinse the curlers thoroughly with tepid water. Remove them carefully and rinse again thoroughly until all the neutralizer is removed. At this point the wig is ready to be set into a particular style, but since the permanent wave could possibly have caused a small amount of damage, the application of a conditioner or normalizer is recommended. One ounce of vinegar in eight ounces of water is a good normalizer.

Falls, Wiglets, Longer Hairpieces, and Spot Curling

The category of falls, wiglets, and longer hairpieces also includes long wigs. On these pieces, end curls only may be desired. In this event, you should roll the hair around the curler only about three to five inches. This procedure will give curl and body to the ends. You may spot curl any section of a wig where you need more body or curl to make your style keep. Necklines that have been cut resulting in stubby ends can be curled for easier and better styling.

Special Problems

Hair tinted with metallic dyes and rinses will discolor when permanent waved; usually it will darken. Observe this change on your test curl. DO NOT permanent wave if the test shows this discoloration. Remember: The hair in most human-hair goods, especially those pieces manufactured in the Orient, are bleached and then dyed to the various shades. The hair is not always bleached to the same stage of porosity. Even in the same wig or hairpiece, the porosity will vary to a great extent. This is one reason that wig hair can be overprocessed so easily.

Protective Measures

For each cold wave, you should either wear rubber gloves or use a protective cream preparation to protect your skin from chemical action of the cold waving solutions. In rinsing the neutralizer from the curlers, rinse the wig cap very thoroughly also, so that no cold waving solution is left in the cap to cause chemical reactions to your customer's skin.

EQUIPMENT USED IN COLD WAVING

1. Cold wave curlers
2. Endpapers
3. Plastic squeeze bottles
4. Dry towels
5. Cold wave solution
6. Rubber gloves or protective cream

EXERCISE

1. What type of hair can be successfully permanent waved? _____

_____

2. What is cold waving?_____

_____

3. What solution strength should be used in permanent waving wigs and hairpieces? _____

_____

4. Why are preliminary test curls necessary before attempting a cold wave on a wig or hairpiece? _____

_____

5. What factors determine the size of the wave or curl pattern? _____

_____

6. Why should no tension be used when wrapping the hair onto the curler? _____

_____

7. When is the waving solution applied? _____

_____

8. How can you determine when the proper curling is completed?

_____

9. How much time should be allowed for neutralizing?_____

_____

10. When is a normalizer used? _____

_____

11. What effect does cold wave solution have on hair treated with metallic dyes or rinses? _____

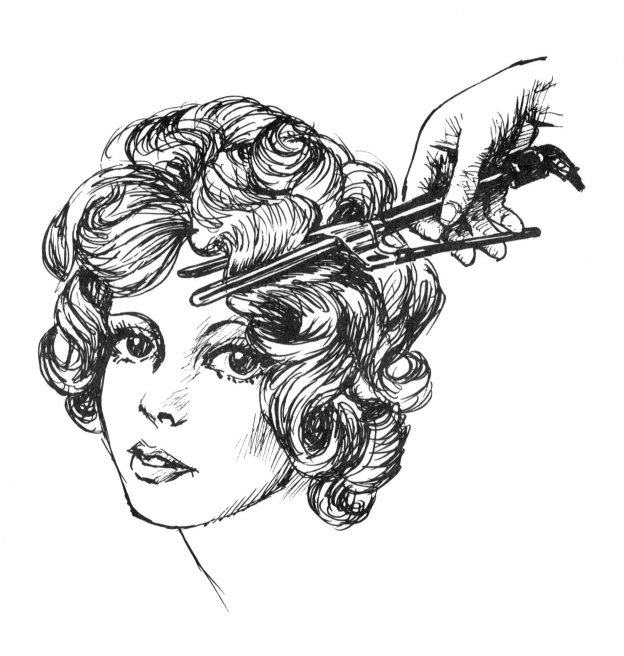

Chapter 9   HOT IRON STYLING

Hot irons are very necessary to the modern wigologist. There are many times that you will do a complete set with them or if a finished hairset is not right you can use them to re-direct the curls so that the customer will like the style. The best irons to use are the ones with a heat control. The heat controlled iron that uses a slight oil vapor is even better. The wigologist that is proficient with hot irons can set any piece in a matter of minutes, let cool, and then comb out. If you use the irons with a slight oil vapor, there is less damage to the hair and a firmer, more lasting set. Hot irons cannot be used on every piece. For example, very blond or over-bleached hair will break or scorch with the use of the irons.

HOW TO USE HOT IRONS

First grip the handle firmly in the palm of your hand, placing your first two fingers over the lower part of the handle so that you can hold the irons firmly and control the curling action with the fingers. Open and close the spoon and barrel of the curling iron several times to practice and get the feel of them, using your little finger for control. Now open and close the iron, moving your wrist from side to side. Practice until you feel you have a good grip and that you can control the opening and closing of the spoon and barrel of the iron.

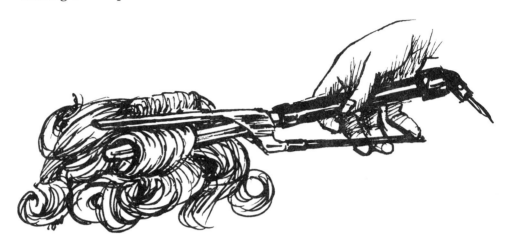

Now block a hairpiece and part off a curl section. Hold the hair straight up with your free hand. Open your iron and place it at the base of the hair, close the barrel and spoon and slide them up to the end of the hair, warming the hair two or three times. Now you are ready to make a curl.

Taking the small curl section you have warmed, you are now ready to curl. Insert the irons approximately one-half inch to one inch from the base. Roll the irons under, using wrist action opening and closing the irons, until the spoon faces the wigologist.

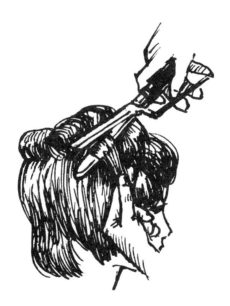

With your free hand catch the ends of the hair, still opening and closing and rolling the irons and keeping them the same distance from the base. Now using wrist action, draw the hair toward the end of the irons.

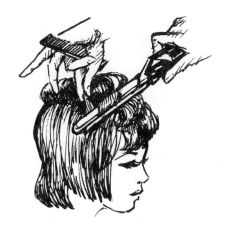

Loop the hair underneath the tips of the irons. Hold your irons tightly, shifting the fingers to the underneath handle, and push the irons forward just a little. By pushing the irons forward and pulling the hair with the free hand, you have formed two loops of your curl, and there is still free hair extending from the iron. Now roll, and open and close the irons, and the ends of the hair will disappear. Roll your irons, hold, pull your irons out and you have formed your first curl.

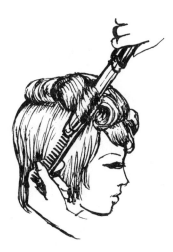

With practice this will become very easy.

EXAMPLES:

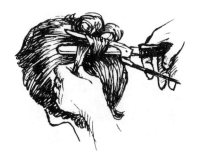 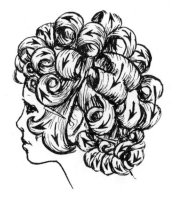

This is only one way to use the irons. There are many versions you will develop as a result of practice with this method. For example, using somewhat the same method, you can make ridge waves, roller curls, and even pin curls. Practice is the only answer to using the hot irons.

ELECTRIC HEAT ROLLING

Heat rolling works very much like the heat irons, but it is done with a set of pre-heated rollers.

EXAMPLE:

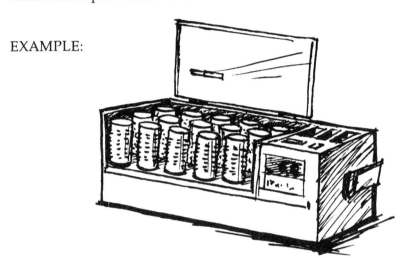

You can set a full wig, hairpiece, or fall with heated rollers. The curl will not be as strong, but the setting method with heat rollers is exactly the same as rolling a wig or hairpiece with rollers. Heat rollers are used effectively in doing "put on's" of hairpieces when the head of hair on which you are placing your piece does not go in the direction you desire. It is simply a quick set.

ELECTRIC HEAT COMBS

Electric heat combs are good to use to straighten out over-curly synthetics, to give hair direction, and to add body. You can even direct curl with a heat comb, similar to the way you would wrap the hair around the curling iron by holding the hair over the barrel. Heat combs are especially good, too, for men's styling.

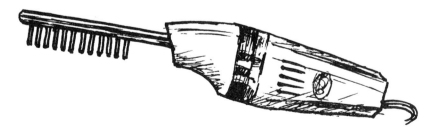

1. What uses can the wigologist find for hot irons?_____

_____

2. Name the parts of the curling irons._____

3. With practice, what different curls can a wigologist make with hot

   irons? _____

4. Describe heat rollers. _____

5. For what are heat rollers used? _____

6. What is a heat comb? _____

7. What are the uses of the heat comb?_____

_____

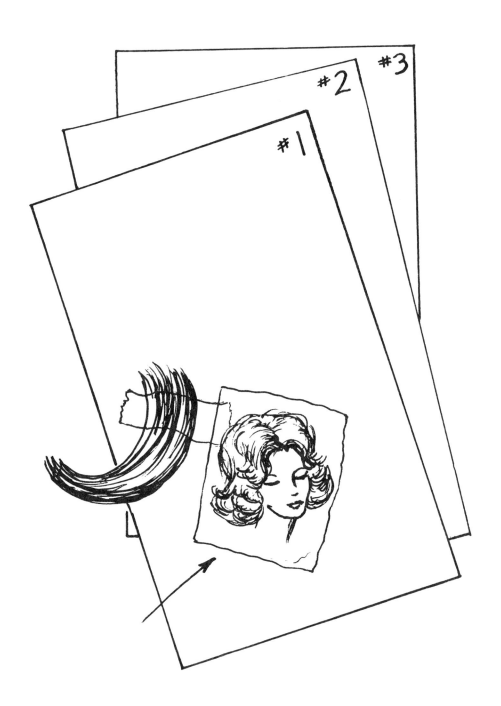

#1

#2

#3

Chapter 10   TICKET SYSTEM

Your ticket system is as important as your customer identification card. First of all, it provides you with proper identification of the hairgoods you are servicing and the style for your customer, and it should remain with this piece at all times during the service process. Whenever a customer leaves a hairpiece with an operator, she should take it immediately to the desk and tag it with the customer ticket. All hairgoods should come through the front desk.

You should have a ticket book in triplicate. When the customer leaves a wig or hairpiece with you, get her name, address, and phone number (should you need to call her with a question pertaining to her wig), date the ticket, describe the hairstyle, and record the date and time she wishes to pick the piece up. At this time, pin one ticket to her wig, one to the case, and give her the third copy. (Note that it is very important that you always price out your tickets, so there will be no question about how much your customer pays for her services.) You then place her pick-up or appointment time in your appointment book. The appointment book should be kept for all customers wishing to have you add a hairpiece or to have a wig put on and adjusted by you. The only way you will be able to keep track of your customers is to use this book.

You now should place the ticketed wig in a bin at your station or in bins provided in the dispensary, organized according to the day the wig is to be picked up.

SAMPLE APPOINTMENT BOOK

DATE	YEAR		DATE	YEAR	
TIME	OPERATOR NAME	OPERATOR NAME	OPERATOR NAME	OPERATOR NAME	OPERATOR NAME
8:00					
8:30					
9:00					
9:30					
10:00					
10:30					
11:00					
11:30					
12:00					
12:30					
1:00					
1:30					
2:00					
2:30					
3:00					
3:30					
4:00					

Each appointment is entered in the appointment book for the time chosen by the customer, and if any additional time is going to be needed, mark it out when the appointment is booked. If a customer does not show up for her appointment, her name should be circled or marked through so you will know her ticket will not be in the day's receipts.

TICKETING PROCEDURE

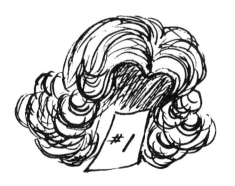

Customer wig is tagged with ticket #1 as it is brought into the salon.

Customer case or styrofoam head is tagged with ticket #2.

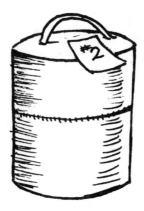

Customer leaves with ticket #3.

Ticket stays with wig during cleaning and drying.

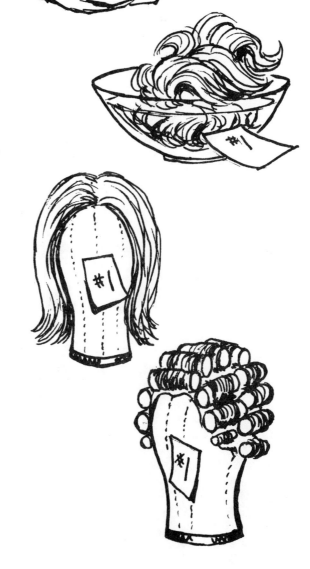

Ticket remains with wig during during blocking.

Ticket stays with wig while wig is set and dried.

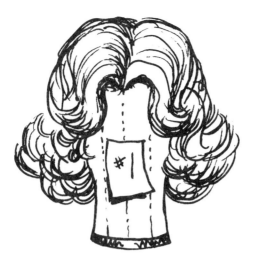

Ticket is attached to combed wig, ready for customer pick-up.

If your customer does not leave a case, place two tickets on her wig. This will indicate to you that she has not left a case, and if she had forgotten and thought her case was there, you have proof with the two tickets. The ticket must remain with the wig at all times; pin the wig on the block and pin the ticket securely on the front of the block.

When your customer picks up the wig, you put it on her head for the finishing touches. Then get her case, put both tickets together, place one on the spindle, collect her money. Dispose of the ticket that was attached to the case. This ticketing procedure is the only way by which you can be sure that you will not lose the customer's hairpiece.

TRIPLICATE COPY

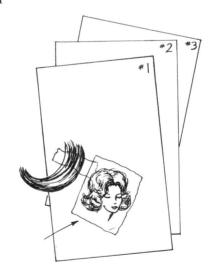

1. How many copies are suggested for a customer service ticket? _____

2. Why do you need three copies of a service ticket? 1. _____
    2. _____ 3. _____

3. Why should you place the customer's phone number on her service
    ticket? _____

4. Is it important to price a ticket before a customer leaves her hair-
    goods with you? Why? _____
    _____

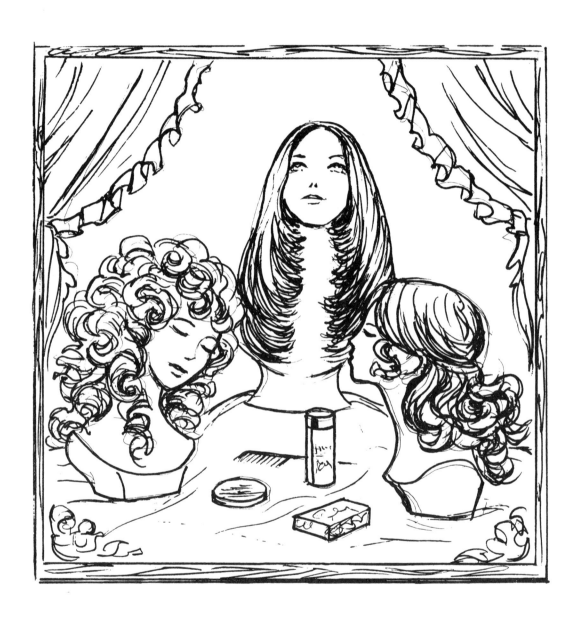

Chapter 11 SALES AND SALESMANSHIP

Selling is the link between the product and the need of the customer. A good salesman will produce a satisfied customer, not just a sale for profit. The sale is not ended with the receipt of the money but should be the beginning of a successful relationship between the salesman and the satisfied customer.

Sales are the lifeblood of your business or the shop you are employed in. Consider this: If you do not sell wigs and hairpieces, there will be nothing to service. Selling to the customer is your business. It is where you build your clientele and produce the products with which you work. Every part of your technical training must be sold to the customer. To become a good salesman, with new merchandise or the re-sell of your services, depends on your eagerness and ability to develop a smooth, complete sales approach with which you feel relaxed and confident.

The selling of wigs and hairpieces is a unique type of sales because of the personal knowledge you must have of your customer and the fact that your judgment will do much to guide the customer's decision. With practice you will learn to handle specific situations associated with these sales. Often, for example, the customer may come to you having a wrong selection in mind. She may ask for a certain type of piece to do a specific style. You know that this piece will not do what is desired and would be a wrong choice for her. You must then guide the customer to make the proper selection of the correct piece for her needs. Another situation will involve interpretation and fulfillment of the customer's needs. There are times when the customer does not know what she wants except that she needs or desires extra hair. It is your job to determine what she needs and for what purpose. To determine her purpose and need, you would ask her where she intends to wear this wig or hairpiece, how much she will depend upon it, and how much head coverage she expects. Knowing the answers to these questions will enable you to advise her in a professional manner. A final step in the selling of hairpieces involves training the customer. Once the sale has been completed and the piece is styled, you should explain to the customer how to care for the wig or hairpiece. Show her how to put it on, how to take it off, and different placements of the hairpiece on the head to achieve different styles and effects. Put the piece on the customer the first time and explain the procedure. Make sure that she is satisfied, because if she is you may be assured of her repeat business.

The following list should help you develop a competent sales procedure.

1. Have a positive attitude, confident and without doubt.
2. Greet your prospective customer pleasantly. Smile, and ask how you may be of service to her.
3. Find out what her needs are. Why does she need this additional hair? For social reasons, functional purposes, sports, medical reasons?
4. Determine the amount the customer is willing to spend for the merchandise. Give her several price ranges to select from, and explain the quality of each.
5. Show her merchandise within her price range, but do not be fearful of showing her merchandise *over* the price range she has quoted to you. Give her a choice from the price range she has quoted and from a price range above what she has quoted, but never below.
6. When showing merchandise, include the following points in your presentation:
    (a) Do not confuse the customer with too many pieces.
    (b) Explain the quality and make of each piece.
    (c) Explain the uses of the different pieces.
    (d) Give the advantages of each piece.
7. Encourage the customer to ask questions concerning the merchandise. Answer all of her questions, keep all your answers simple. Try to explain care in a methodical manner. Leave her with the thought that if she has a difficulty later, you will be available to help her.
8. After the customer has selected a piece of merchandise, try the piece on her. Check the color and the style very carefully. Check the size, for alteration purposes.

9.　Write a ticket and make an appointment for the time your customer will pick up her new wig or hairpiece. Take a deposit or payment on the merchandise she has selected.

10.　Follow up your sale. Be ready and available to put the merchandise on your customer at pick-up time. Be prepared to make any alterations necessary to fulfill your sales promise to your customer. Make sure she is satisfied and will return.

Most important, relax and be yourself. Anyone will detect tenseness and phoniness. The good first impression you give her is the one she will expect next time, and the one she will return to!

MERCHANDISE

Every shop has something to sell, and it should be displayed the very best it possibly can be at all times. If you can help with the merchandise when you are not busy, *do so*. All display merchandise must be kept neat and orderly. Knowing the stock in the shop will help you sell it. Keep all hair goods brushed and looking neat and clean. They do not need to be styled, simply displayed nicely. Keeping a sample of your work on the shelf by your station will show customers what the styled pieces look like. Also, finished wigs of your customers will serve as a display of your own personal work. Your shop owner may handle products that re-condition wigs or hair-holding sprays, wave sets, and other products pertaining to hair; display these at your station with his permission.

Even the smallest spaces can produce a revenue; let's make money and sell!

YOUR STATION

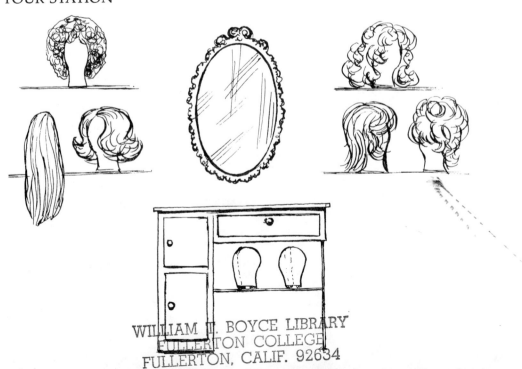

EXERCISE

1. What is selling? _____

2. What is the importance of selling wigs and hairpieces? _____

   _____

3. Why is the selling of wigs and hairpieces unique?_____

   _____

4. What things are basic to the sales procedure?

   A. _____   F. _____

   B. _____   G. _____

   C. _____   H. _____

   D. _____   I. _____

   E. _____   J. _____

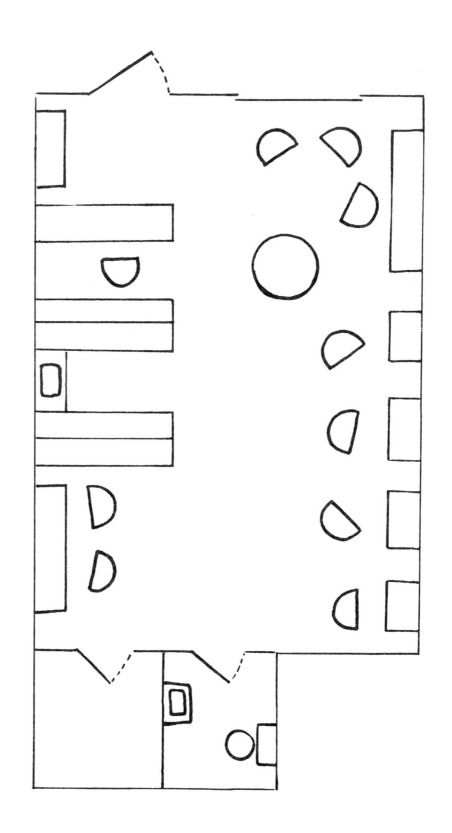

Chapter 12 BUSINESS MANAGEMENT

LOCATION

In the selection of the physical location of your wig salon, special consideration should be given to the area, the traffic flow, visibility from street side, the general attractiveness of the center or surrounding area, parking area, density of population, and overall average income of the area. You should certainly satisfy yourself that the area in which you plan to invest in your wig salon will support the business and that the store you have selected will be attractive and large enough in which to do business.

LEASE OR RENTAL OF STORE SPACE

For your mutual protection, you and your landlord should agree on lease terms, not only on the amount of rent you will pay, but also on exactly what his responsibilities are, especially regarding:

1. Plumbing or electrical failure
2. Store and parking area maintenance, including lights
3. Painting and redecorating

4.   Glass breakage
5.   Liability insurance
6.   Exclusiveness of your type of business
7.   Leasehold improvements

If you are moving into a new building or a new center, have a signed agreement between you and your landlord stating exactly what part of the construction you are responsible for, especially regarding:

1.   Partitions
2.   Restrooms
3.   Plumbing
4.   Flooring
5.   Store front
6.   Lighting fixtures
7.   Architectural fees
8.   Painting
9.   Air conditioning

Of course, these examples do not cover everything, but using them as a basis for discussion with your landlord will save you many misunderstandings, headaches, and unnecessary expense later.

There are no rules regarding the length of leases. You must bear in mind that you are going into business with the desire and attitude that you will be successful, so don't let a five-year lease frighten you. Probably the best way to protect yourself in your location is to request a term of three to five years with one or two options to renew. A landlord will usually be receptive to this request, especially in centers that contain larger stores. Review your lease with your attorney so that he may help you understand it more fully.

LICENSES

In almost every town and state there are licenses and permits that you must obtain before you can legally operate your salon. Your attorney and accountant can advise you as to your specific needs, but they will usually consist of some or all of the following:

1.   State store license. Apply to the State Comptroller in your state capital.
2.   City or county store license. Apply at your City Hall and County Court House.
3.   Health inspection certificate. This is controlled usually at the city or county level.

4. State license for wig salon. Apply to the State Cosmetology Commission at your state capital.

5. Individual operator's license. Apply to the State Cosmetology Commission at your state capital.

6. Sales tax permit. Apply to the State Comptroller at your state capital.

7. Employer's identification number. Apply to the Internal Revenue Service Regional Office.

INSURANCE AND LIABILITY

The extent of your liability and obligations to your customers and to the general public should be discussed jointly with your attorney and insurance agent. There are certain types of insurance that are necessary for you to have. In most instances, they are:

1. Premises liability, including general or public liability. This protects you against any claims that may arise from the injury to your customers while in or about your salon. This will include falling over furniture, tripping over wires, or slipping on the floors. Caution: Make certain your coverage includes the sidewalk as well as the inside of your salon.

2. Sign insurance. Usually signs are not covered in your general public liability, nor in your regular hazard policy. Special consideration is to be given to protect yourself against claims in the event that your sign is blown down or falls to the ground. Also, you will want to protect yourself against the expense of replacing the sign.

3. Bailee liability. Wigs and merchandise goods left in your care by customers are covered only by a Bailee Liability policy. This will cover theft, fire, or other accidental damage.

4. Insurance against fire and other hazards. This will protect you against the loss of your equipment, furniture, fixtures, and supplies by fire, wind storms and water damages. Usually this coverage does not include burglary and theft.

5. Burglary insurance. This type of coverage will protect you against the loss of merchandise (other than customer wigs), fixtures, and equipment from theft by burglary. Remember that this insurance does not necessarily cover customers' property, so check closely.

6. Workmen's compensation. This insurance is required by law to cover your employees in the event of accidental injury while on the job.

Insurance laws vary from state to state. Your attorney and insurance agent can advise you of what is required and what each classification covers. Satisfy yourself that you have what you want and that you understand what you are buying. One insurance term to understand is co-insurance. Basically, it means that if you do not insure for the full value, you, yourself, share in the losses proportionately to the extent that the amount of insurance falls short of a specified percentage of the value of the property. This could prove costly to you in the event of a loss. Understand this term fully.

BOOKKEEPING AND RECORD KEEPING

If at all possible, you should have a competent accountant assist you in designing a bookkeeping and tax records system to fit your needs. Your basic bookkeeping needs are fairly simple, and a system can be devised so that you can handle it yourself on a daily basis. An office supply store can furnish you with bookkeeping materials to fit your needs. This will consist of a ledger-size book that has step-by-step instructions and all the necessary pre-printed forms you will need. In it, there will be a section for:

1. Daily sales, totaled weekly, then monthly.
2. Daily expense, totaled weekly, then monthly.
3. Payroll records, totaled quarterly for tax purposes.
4. Summaries of sales and expenses, total monthly, then quarterly.
5. Profit and loss statements, showing you your profit or loss.

These pre-printed bookkeeping systems are complete, and if used correctly, with postings being made daily without fail, will provide you with a very good picture of what and how your business is doing. You will have totals on a breakdown of expenses that can be analyzed in making decisions with regard to changes in your operation. Knowing where every cent comes from and goes to will give you a clearer overall picture.

The type of form on page 109 will give you your daily and weekly sales figures. Of course, the form can be redesigned to give an even more complete picture, if desired, such as breaking the sales figure down into more specific departments or categories, showing each individual operator's sales, wig service, etc. The daily report form is designed for three distinct, timesaving purposes: (1) to give you an accurate picture of your day's activity; (2) to allow you to keep a close daily account of your cash; and (3) to provide information that must be included in your overall bookkeeping system, with regard to total sales, individual operator sales, sales tax, cash payouts, and bank deposits. This should be done in accordance with instructions from your accountant or the instruction sheet accompanying the bookkeeping system you may purchase.

SAMPLE DAILY OPERATING REPORT

DAY AND DATE	TOTAL SALES			TOTAL SALES #1	SALES TAX #2	PAID OUT CASH #3	OTHER DISCOUNTS #4	TOTAL 1+2 −3−4	TOTAL BANK DEPOSITS	OVER / UNDER
	HAIR GOODS	BOUTIQUE	SERVICE							
Mon										
Tue										
Wed										
Thur										
Fri										
Sat										
Sun										
Total										

Because of the necessity for accuracy, your bookkeeping system should be audited regularly by an accountant. If quarterly audits are made prior to preparing and completing your year-end tax reports, any errors can be corrected at that time.

OPERATING STATEMENTS

An operating statement, also called a profit and loss statement, is of vital importance to you at the end of every month. This statement will give you a complete picture of your month's activities, sales, and expenses. The operating statement should include such information on a year to date basis. Information from your daily reports posted into the general ledger, along with postings from your check stubs covering your payrolls and accounts payable, are totaled into monthly totals, and these totals are posted to the operating statement. A typical form should include the following:

OPERATING STATEMENT OF PROFIT OR LOSS

INCOME
  Sales _____
    Hairgoods _____
    Boutique _____
  Service _____
TOTAL INCOME _____

EXPENSES

Payroll and commissions	_____
Payroll and other tax	_____
Merchandise for resale	_____
Laundry service	_____
Equipment repairs	_____
Rent	_____
Insurance	_____
Utilities and telephone	_____
Advertising	_____
Operating supplies	_____
Other expenses	_____
TOTAL EXPENSES	_____
TOTAL INCOME	_____
TOTAL EXPENSES	_____
PROFIT [OR LOSS]	_____

PHYSICAL DESIGN AND LAYOUT OF SALON

The actual physical design of your salon depends on its size and shape, on your own personal taste and preferences, and, of course, on the amount of investment capital available. Keep in mind, however, that you must allow for:

1. Sales and display areas.
2. Work or styling areas.
3. Customer service areas.

These are actually three separate areas that may overlap. However, your work area should be closed off from the other areas, and customers should not have access to it. Care should be taken that there are no exposed obstacles such as wire, furniture, roller trays, dryers, or debris on the floor that could possibly cause a painful or even serious accident to your customers. Keep in mind that you want to provide a clean and pleasant facility for your customers and employees as well. Have a place for everything and keep everything in its proper place. Display your merchandise in as attractive and appealing a manner as possible, and provide comfort, safety, and service for your customers while they are in your salon.

SAMPLE FLOOR PLAN FOR WIG SALON

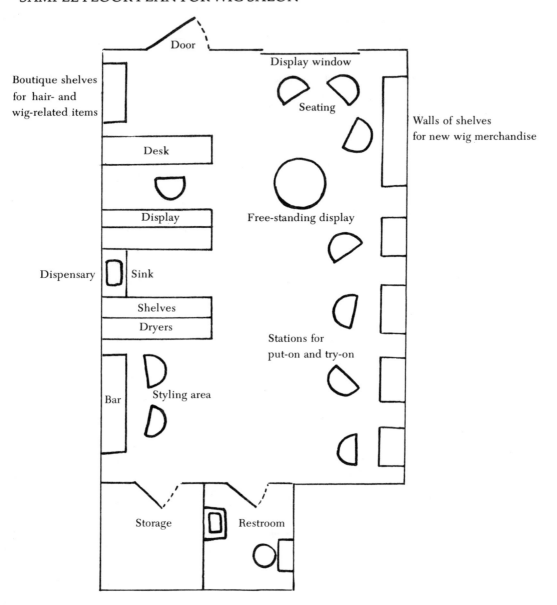

Sales and Display Area

The sales and display area is where your merchandise is displayed for sale. It is where you make your initial contact with your customer. Your merchandise should be displayed in the most attractive and appealing manner possible.

Work or Styling Areas

The styling area is where the service work is done. It should be equipped with the following equipment and supplies:

1. Formica counters with mirrors for each styling station
2. A wig block clamp at each station
3. A drawer or covered container for sanitized brushes and combs, razor, and scissors
4. Sufficient rollers, clippies, and tee pins to fulfill the work schedule
5. Extra canvas blocks
6. Dispensary sink for wetting and color work
7. Large, box dryers for drying wigs
8. Closed waste can and towel bins
9. Operating supplies including wig spray set, setting lotion, various coloring products, and any other items required in your services

Customer Service Area

In this area you present your service customer with her styled and serviced hairpiece. It may also double as a sales and demonstration area. The area is equipped with the following equipment used to put the hairpiece on the customer.

1. Swivel chair or chairs
2. Large mirrors, facing the swivel chairs
3. A drawer or closed containers for sanitized brushes, combs, scissors, and razors

Remember to utilize your space to your best advantage, keeping it uncluttered and smooth-working. Proper design can save you much supervising time and many unnecessary steps, and it will afford your customers pleasant surroundings when they patronize your salon.

ADVERTISING

With the many forms of advertising available, it is difficult to decide just where your advertising money should be spent. Many factors must be considered before you settle on an advertising program for your business. Listed here are some of these factors:

1. Your location with regard to your possible selling area
2. The population density of this area

3. The daily traffic that is already available

4. Income brackets and affluence of the area

5. Your advertising budget

6. Your "slow" and "busy" days

7. Seasons

8. The availability of local area newspapers

9. The impact you want to make and image you wish to project

There are many methods of attracting buyers to your salon. Inquiry, experimentation and the past experience of yourself and others will help you decide on the most effective methods.

Newspaper

Citywide newspaper advertising is generally very expensive, especially if you are located in a large city. However, there are usually local, area newspapers serving small areas of large cities. Quite often the advertising rates of these limited circulation newspapers are within the reach of a salon serving the same general area.

Direct Mail

Direct mail has proven to be a very effective and economical advertising method for businesses of all types and sizes. Mailing lists should be carefully chosen. One of the best sources is your own card file, where you have all of your customers listed. You can compile your own mailing list or purchase lists from direct mail advertising agents. Of course, these direct mail agents can handle the whole program for you, preparing your mailing, addressing letters or flyers, and seeing that they are mailed.

Radio

Radio spot advertising expense varies with the area, time of day, and length of the spot. Radio advertising is usually most effective in a saturation situation or for long-range identification. Costs generally are expensive, but response is usually good, especially in a saturation program. Your choice of the particular station or stations on which to run your advertising depends on several factors, such as (1) the type of audience you want to reach; (2) the area from which you want to pull your prospective customers; and (3) your radio advertising budget.

Television

Television is usually very effective, but also very costly. Large-volume salons or chains can utilize television advertising despite its expense because of the effectiveness of advertising in this media.

PERSONNEL SELECTION AND ADMINISTRATION

The general rule for staffing a salon, of course, is to hire the best people available and give them the opportunity to make the maximum amount of salary your salon can afford. First, determine the number and type of employees you will need, such as sales people, wig stylists, colorists, comb out artists, and helpers. When you decide your needs and hold interviews with prospective employees, the following steps should be taken:

1. Obtain each applicant's full name, address, and telephone number.
2. Determine the amount of specific training that can be applied to the position you are filling.
3. Determine and check on the applicant's experience with previous employers. Ask the employer about the individual's work habits, proficiency, ability to get along with customers and other employees, general attitude, and absenteeism.
4. Outline for the applicant exactly what your job opening is, explaining in detail what the duties and responsibilities are, and what the specific working days and hours will be. Have these all understood.
5. Explain exactly and thoroughly the salary the employee will receive and on which day or date he can expect to be paid. If you work by commission or piece work, outline exactly how the employee's pay is determined.

Your ultimate aim, of course, is to operate your salon on a profitable basis, take care of your customers, and maintain a happy working atmosphere for your employees.

EXERCISE

1. Why is the location of your salon so important? _____
_____

2. Why is it advisable for you to review a business lease with your attorney? _____

3. Where would you apply for a state license for a wig salon? _____
_____

4. Where would you apply for a sales tax permit? _____
_____

5. Why must you have workmen's compensation? _____
_____

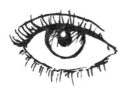
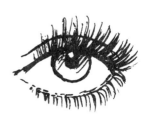
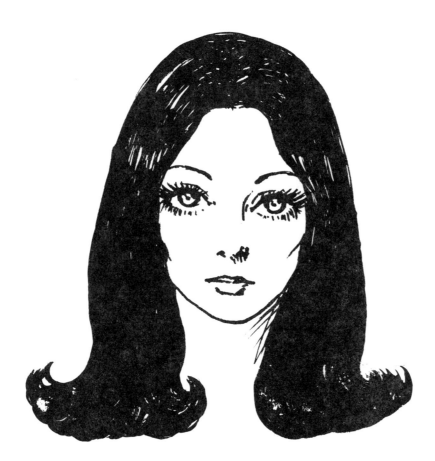

Chapter 13 EYELASH STYLING

Women have always been concerned about the appearance of their eyes. They have used eyeliner, shadows, and false eyelashes, but now they can have the most beautiful, natural look of all with the application of permanent, singularly applied eyelashes. These lashes are made of synthetic fiber; they have permanent curl and will not react to the weather. They are a beautiful frame to enhance the eye and with them you can look good even without makeup. This is one of the best selling points that you can offer.

SUPPLIES

The supplies you will need for a professional eyelash service are these:

1. Trays of synthetic eyelashes from your local supply house. These come in four lengths in both brown and black. The lengths are extra short (referred to as lowers), shorts, mediums, and longs.
2. Special eye makeup remover and lash cleaner.
3. Special eyelash glue, clear and dark.

4. Eyelash glue solvent.

5. Special surgical tweezers, cotton swabs, sterilizer solution for tweezers, scissors, eyelash brush, and hand mirror.

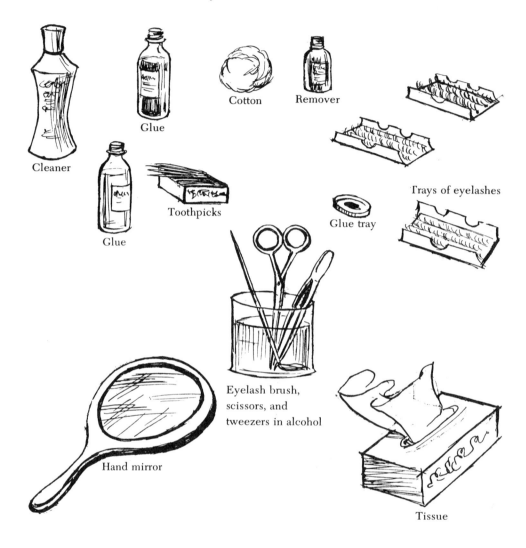

STYLING

The Natural Look

The natural look is achieved by using the short eyelashes combined with the underneath lash. This style will simply thicken the customer's own lashes.

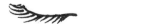

The Fashion Look

The customer may still want a natural look but prefer a longer, more luxurious lash. In this case, you will want to make her lashes appear thicker and longer than her own. This effect is achieved by a heavy application of short and medium length lashes.

 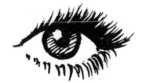

Special Effects

There are women who want a special, more dramatic effect from their lashes, and they prefer a very long, luxurious lash. To achieve this style, use a combination of all lengths or use all long lashes. Customers who want this special effect will sometimes want underneath lashes applied also.

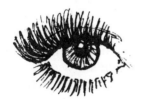 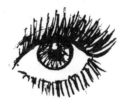

Checkpoints

Look at your customer's natural lashes. In most cases, there will be more than enough natural straight lashes to which to affix all of the lashes required for any desired styling. If the customer's lashes are sparse and she wants a heavy eye tab, you must use corrective tabbing which we will discuss later in this chapter.

You can apply eyelashes to customers who wear contact lenses or eyeglasses, but a little special care is required. If your customer wears contact lenses, ask her to remove them, while you apply the lashes, to reduce tearing. You must also determine the correct *length* of lashes for people who wear eyeglasses. Do this by taking the longest length of lash that you are going to use and place it in the center of the eye. Ask your customer to put on her glasses. If the lash does not touch the lens, it is safe to proceed with this length.

EXAMPLE:

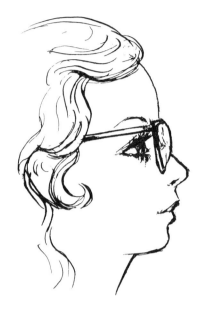

POSITIONING

The position of your customer is important in the eye tabbing process. The stylist works behind the customer at all times, except in the removal process and when the underneath lashes are being applied. The customer should rest in a reclining chair that positions her head at a comfortable working height. Her face should be well-lighted. Her eyes should be open, looking downward at a 45° angle. This will make it easier for you to see her natural lashes.

EXAMPLE:

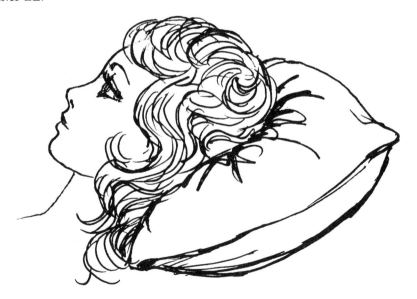

APPLICATION STEPS

1. Since the eyelashes come in trays and the tips are glued to prevent spilling, you must pull them out gently to avoid tearing them apart. Loosen the eyelash first, then pull near the base with tweezers, and draw it loose.

EXAMPLE:

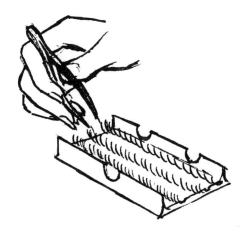

2. Now that you have the lash out of the tray, holding it with your tweezers, dip the bulb end into the glue. Place an amount of glue about the size of a pinhead on the bulb end of the eyelash. Use the clear and the dark glue in most applications. The dark glue accents and the clear leaves a more natural appearance.

EXAMPLE:

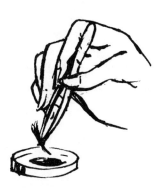

3. You are now ready to start and should select a starting point slightly off center, since this seems to help control the tear flow. Now, you can begin to place your eyelash pattern. It is best to begin with the left eye to prevent brushing the right eye with your hand after it is completed. Work from left to right.

4. After dipping the eyelash in the glue, brush the natural lash with the glue half-way down the lash, and then place the artificial lash on top of the natural lash. The eyelash and the glue will bind together. If the

eyelash should turn, you must hold it into place for a few seconds. Even though the glue and the lash bind instantly, it will take several hours for the glue to set permanently.

EXAMPLE:

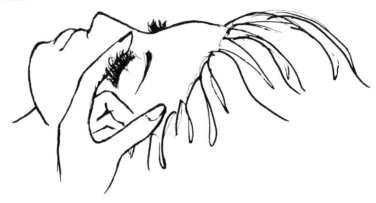

5. The corner lashes are the most difficult to place. You must take the finger of your free hand, use it to hold your customer's eyelid taut, and place the lash to fan out to the natural contour of her eye. Hold her eye open for a few seconds so that the glue will not get on her lower lashes and bind the uppers and lowers together.

EXAMPLE:

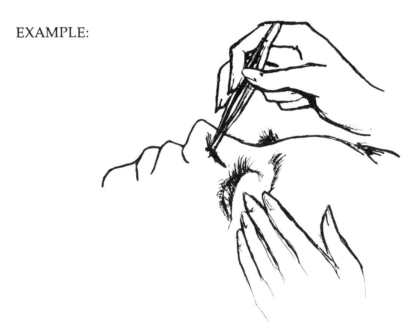

6. The placement of the lower lashes is an additional service. Beautiful as they may be, they will not stay on as long as the uppers because the natural skin oils will loosen the glue after a week causing the added lash to fall off. Be sure to explain this fact to your customer. To place the the lower lashes, you should sit in front of the customer. Ask her to look

up and using the underneath length only, pick up the lash with your tweezers, place it in the glue, run the glue down her natural lash, and then place the underneath lash. Ask your customer to keep her eyes open for a few minutes to give the glue time to harden.

EXAMPLE:

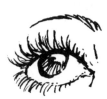 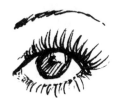

THE USE OF EYELASH REMOVER

Sometimes it is necessary to remove the eyelash after the glue is set. Do not try to pull the eyelashes off with the tweezers as you will also pull your customer's own natural lashes out. Use the following procedure: Have your customer sit up and face you. Place a tissue or an eye pad under her eyelashes with the eyes closed. Using an artist-type brush saturated with the eyelash remover, brush gently until the lash glue dissolves and the lash comes off on the tissue or pad.

EXAMPLE:

Customer sits upright and faces operator for eyelash removal

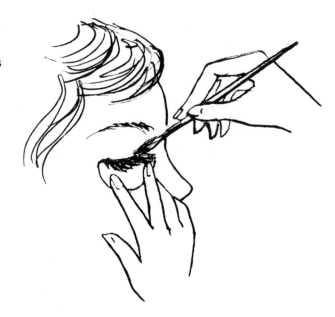

PROBLEMS AND EXPLANATIONS

ALLERGY. If a customer says her eyes are extremely sensitive to allergies, you should place only a couple of lashes on her eye and wait 24 hours. Then if no adverse reaction occurs, proceed with the eye tab.

CLEANING.   Before you start an eye tab on a customer, you must make absolutely certain that all makeup and mascara is removed and that the *lashes are dry*. Take a brush and straighten out all of the customer's lashes. If you take special precautions in cleaning, you will have a better, firmer tab.

TEARING.   Working around the eye area may cause tearing even though you may not touch the lid with the glue. Explain to your customer that this is a perfectly natural occurrence and that the glue is of surgical nature. Note: Tearing out of the eye you are not working on is caused by apprehension. When you begin working on the eye that is tearing, the tearing will stop. Be sure to re-dry the eye before you start working. If the tearing really becomes a problem, work from one eye to the other.

HEAT.   Be sure to schedule your eyelash customer after her hair has been dried. Heat affects the drying of the eyelash glue and the heat of the dryer may cause freshly applied lashes to fall off.

PROBLEM LASH STYLING.   There will be times when your customer does not have enough eyelashes of her own yet wants a heavy lash look. This is really no problem. Synthetic lashes have about four hairs attached to each bulb. Simply take your fingers and spread the lash, gluing one side to the side of your customer's natural lash and the other side to the next closest natural lash. The fan shape will make a base on which to glue additional artificial lashes. You may fan and tab the eye as heavily as the customer requests.

THE CURLY LASH.   If your customer's natural lashes are too curly, you must glue the artificial lashes to the side of the natural lashes. This method will produce a more uniform look than if you glued on top of the curly lash.

EXAMPLE:

Glue to side of
the eyelash that
is very curly

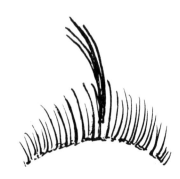

SERVICE

The initial eye tab will take about twenty to thirty minutes. Note: The artificial lashes last as long as your natural lashes, which replace themselves about every six weeks to two months. This does not mean that all of the lashes fall out at one time, but that only a few a week do so, so your customer will require service of a couple of lashes every week or two. This will keep the eyes looking good at all times. Remember, it is better for you and your customer to do the replacement every week so that it will take only a couple of minutes each time. If your customer is going on a vacation for a few weeks the lashes that do come out will hardly be noticed. Tell her not to worry, but simply to see you when she comes back.

The eyelash service is a very good business and if the customer knows that she must make an appointment for this service, it will not interfere with your regular routine. Always have your lash tray set up with the essentials to accommodate your customer's needs. This will save valuable time.

Make sure that your customer is happy with her eyes and if, as time goes by, she wants the eyelash style changed, all you have to do is add various lengths or even remove a few lashes and change them.

Be sure to instruct your customer in the care of her new lashes. Tell her to cleanse them as normal, but not to use cleanser on the eyelid. Use the special eyelash cleanser to remove makeup around the eye, since heavy creams will dissolve the glue. The application of the artificial eyelashes does not hinder your customer's normal activities; she can wash her face, splash it with water, swim, and so forth.

This new service is a very profitable innovation to the beauty field and will increase your personal income and enlarge your customer clientele.

EXERCISE

1. What is eye tabbing? _____
2. What fiber is used most in eye tabbing and why? _____

_____

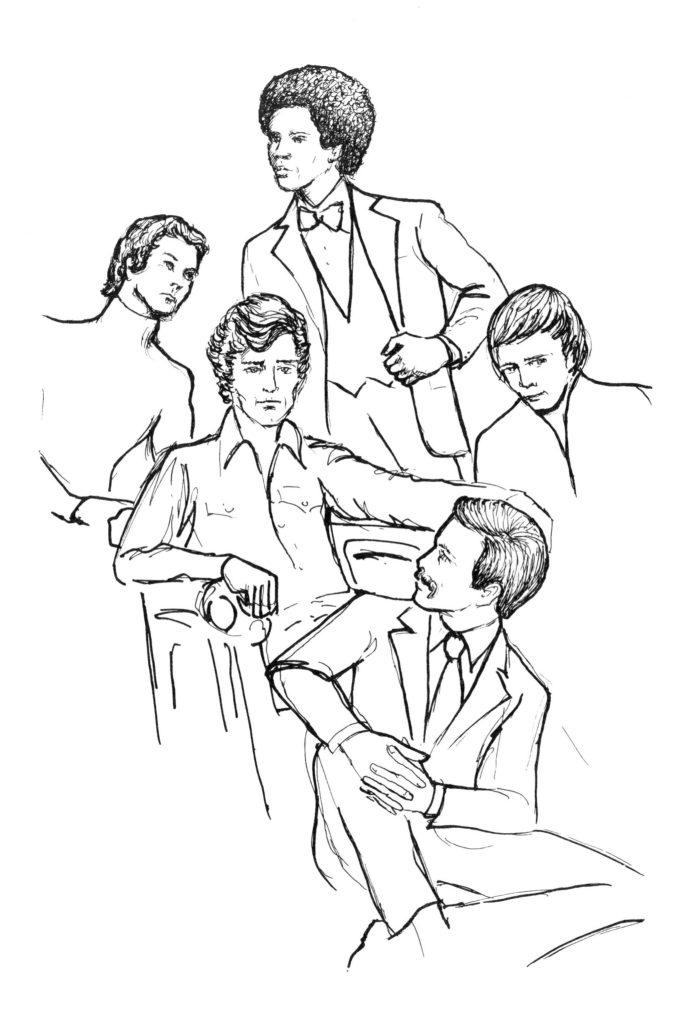

Chapter 14   MEN'S STYLING

HISTORY OF MEN'S WIGS

The apprenticeship of wigmaking that was passed down from one generation to the next is now almost extinct. The tools used even today by the few remaining wigmakers are still rather crude. Modern machines and synthetic fibers, with the aid of mass production and department store outlets, have pushed the small independent wigmaker to the side.

Yet the purchasers of men's wigs require the services of a professional wigologist for cutting, fitting, styling, cleaning, and general wearing tips.

IDENTIFICATION OF MEN'S WIGS

Marketing of mass produced men's hairgoods has produced a new field for the wigologist. Chapter 1 outlined the different types of wigs available and the most desired cuts and styles of these wigs. These divisions (human hair, hand-made; human hair, machine-made; synthetic, hand-made; synthetic, machine-made; synthetic, semi-machine-made) also apply to men's hairgoods.

You will want to keep a customer identification card on each of your male customers.

CUSTOMER IDENTIFICATION CARD

Date:

NAME_____   PHONE   Home_____

                                           Office_____

ADDRESS_____

CITY_____ STATE_____ ZIP_____

HEAD MEASUREMENTS   STYLING INSTRUCTIONS

COLOR SAMPLES   SPECIAL INSTRUCTIONS
Front:
SIDES:
BACK:

Take all of the information necessary, then proceed with the cutting, sizing, and care of this wig or hairpiece.

Sizing skills are vital when fitting a man's head because the closeness of the hairstyle makes it impossible to cover any flaws in the base. In altering a pre-cut stretch wig or a factory wig, you will find that the temple area of the foundation often extends too far on the temple, and this must be cut back in order to produce a more natural hairline.

EXAMPLE:

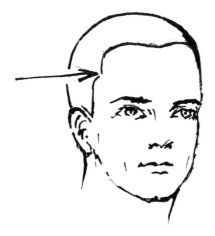

Such an alteration may be accomplished by a V-shaped incision to fit the more natural growth of your customer's hairline. This incision must be re-bound carefully to make it lie flat.

ALTERATION OF WOMAN'S WIG FOR USE AS A MEN'S HAIRPIECE

Man's Wig Cap

Long ear flaps
Back flap

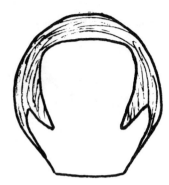

Woman's Wig Cap

Short ear flaps

Round back; base with elastic
strap

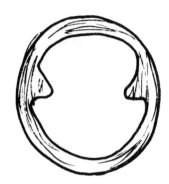

Remove the elastic straps from the nape area of a woman's wig. Make
two, flat vertical darts at the nape area.

EXAMPLE:

Flat dart

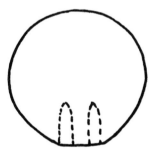

Sew a piece of wide elastic (½ to ¾ inch elastic) to form a square flap at
the back of the wig.

EXAMPLE:

Square elastic

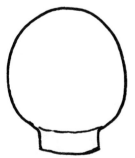

Alterations on *any* head—male or female—are the same; please refer to Chapter 2 on sizing. After the wig fits perfectly and the alterations are made, the customer and the wigologist will decide on the style.

SAMPLE CUT

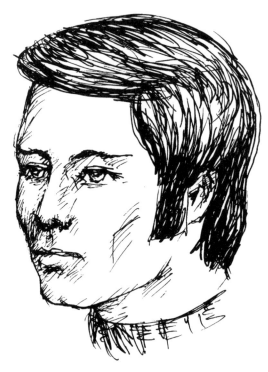

CUTTING METHODS

On synthetic hair, use only your thinning shears, fine tooth, both for length and bulk. Finish the cut with regular cutting shears. Note: Remember that synthetics stretch and spur if cut with a razor. They also look very blunt and chopped if cut with regular cutting shears. On human hair, you should do a razor cut and finish it with regular scissors. When styling a man's wig, it is more desirable to get the exact shape by cutting it on the customer's head, in order to conform the shape with the nape hair and sideburns.

In combing a styled wig, an electric heat blower comb may be used to direct and fluff the hair, and it can also help produce a controlled amount of curl.

TOUPEES

A toupee is a patch of false hair similar to a hairpiece. It is used to fill in an area of the hair where there is baldness or to add fullness for a man with thin hair. Toupees vary in size according to the area of the head you want covered.

EXAMPLE:

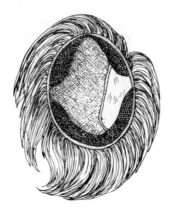

MEASURING FOR A TOUPEE

A. Place plastic wrap on top of the head and mold it to the head's shape.

B. Masking tape is then placed only across area to be covered.

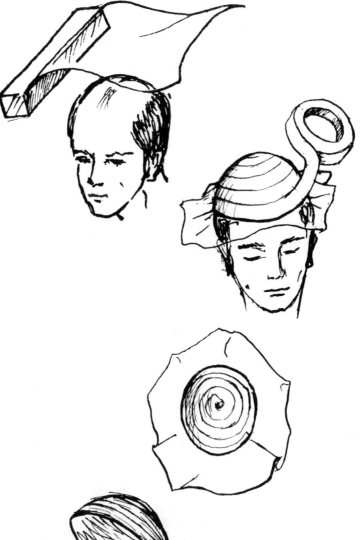

C. Remove the shell of plastic wrap and masking tape from head.

D. Trim the plastic wrap, leaving only the shell of the head imprint.

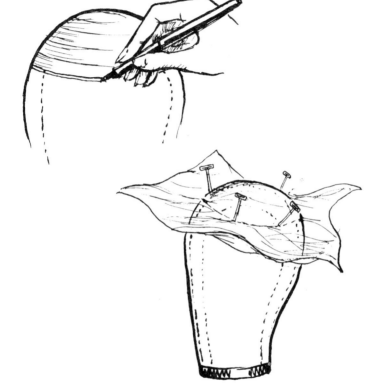

E. Fit the shell to the appropriate block head.

F. Trace the shell shape onto block with a tracing pen.

G. Cut fine mesh material, similar to women's hosiery, to fit this shell drawing.

It is not a general practice for salons to make their own toupees, but to measure the area, make a customer identification card, and take three or four hair samples from different sections of the head to insure a better color match. Take or send this card to a broker or custom wigmaker who will make the toupee. If a pre-cut toupee of lesser quality is desired, the measurements may be transferred to the cap by you. The selection of color is a most important consideration because the hair must blend into the customer's own hair without any color break. You should explain to your customer at this time that he may expect some lightening of color in his toupee if it is human hair, because human hair fades with the sun and the elements. At some time in the future he may need additional color.

Attachment

In order to hold a toupee in place, you must use either glue, such as spirit gum, or tape, whichever you prefer. These may be purchased from supply houses and applied as the manufacturer suggests.

Spirit Gum:

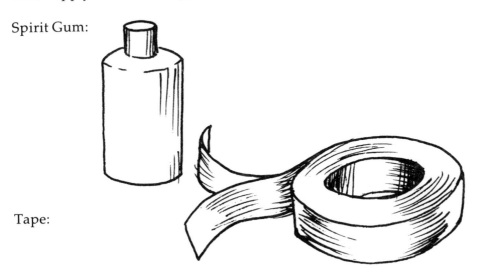

Tape:

EXERCISE

1. What happened to the apprentice wigmaker? _____
   _____

2. Can women's wigs be modified to meet a man's need? _____

3. If a trouble spot arises in a pre-cut stretch wig or factory wig in the
   temple area, what can be done to correct this?_____
   _____

4. Why is it more desirable to cut a man's wig on his head?_____
   _____

5. What is a toupee? _____

6. Do all toupees come in the same size? _____
   _____

7. Name two kitchen products used in measuring for a toupee.
   A. _____   B. _____

8. Why is it necessary to have more than one hair sample for a toupee?
   _____

9. How may a toupee be held in place? _____
   _____

ANSWERS
TO EXERCISES

CHAPTER 1

1. Since 4000 B.C.
2. Wool, palm, silver, and gold.
3. Adornment; medical reasons; for shorter lengths of hair; for longer lengths of hair; vacation or travel.
4. Hand-tied wig: Full coverage
   Man-made wig: Full coverage
   Mini-fall: Swing
   Midi-fall: Flip
   Maxi-fall: Ponytail
   Toppette: Cap style
   Cascade: Curls
   Hair piece, flat base: Filler
   Alura: Full-coverage
5. A machine-stitched strip of hair.
6. Hair cut directly from the head.
7. Hair obtained from combings.
8. Three to five ounces.
9. A wig made of Oriental hair in an Oriental country.

CHAPTER 2

1. Around the head; ear to ear; front to back; temple to temple.
2. No, if the wig is put on the wrong size of block when it is being serviced, the size can be changed.
3. Using tee pins, pin off four measurements on a canvas block.
4. Inside out.
5. When the customer has fine thin hair or will not be letting her hair grow longer.
6. The same color as the inside of the cap.
7. Comfort and styling.
8. No. The cut will not be right.
9. Yes.
10. Six
11. Yes, it should be balanced to the area it will be placed on the head.
12. Tape measure, index card, canvas block, tee pins, vise or clamp, needle and thread, scissors, gold safety pins.

CHAPTER 3

1. Like clothing, it should be cleaned when dirty. This will be about every six to eight weeks if the wig is worn twice a week, every two weeks if it is worn every day.
2. No, it may be cleaned off the block.
3. Brush; immerse in fluid; clean inside of cap; soak three to four minutes; run fingers from base through all hair.
4. Clean inside of cap; brush; block; immerse in fluid; soak; run fingers through hair from base out.
5. All hand-tied pieces.
6. Brush; wet with cold water; clean inside of cap with shampoo and brush; shampoo hair with fingers going through fiber.
7. Dry cleaning solution; glass or porcelain bowls; conditioners; wig or baby shampoo; large-tooth comb; small brush for inside of wig; rubber gloves.

CHAPTER 4

1. To protect your and your customer's health.
2. Microscopic vegetable organisms found everywhere.
3. Heat, disinfectants, ultraviolet rays.
4. 212° Farenheit for 20 minutes.

5. A chemical vapor used to keep objects sanitary.

6. A chemical agent having the power to destroy bacteria.

7. Remove all hair; wash in hot soapy water; immerse in disinfectant; rinse; place in cabinet with ultraviolet rays.

8. In a drawer or cabinet with a fumigant until used.

9. A solution of benzyl benzoate.

10. Unclean wigs are unsanitary, and dirty hair will not style properly.

11. Clean with alcohol or antiseptic.

12. Discard them.

13. With a solution of 70 percent alcohol.

14. With a solution of 70 percent alcohol.

CHAPTER 5

1. Sized for the customer.

2. Regular hair shaping scissors; thinning shears; straight razor; combs.

3. The hair can then be cut systematically, and the result will be a uniform cut.

4. Around the hairline.

5. Front area; temple area; behind the ears.

6. The fall may slip from one side to the other, causing an uneven cut.

7. From as close to the base as possible.

8. It should be held flat with the pressure on the back side of the razor.

9. "More can be taken off"; often "enough cannot be put back on."

CHAPTER 6

1. Base; stem; circle.

2. The width of the wave and its strength.

3. A curl directed toward the face.

4. Direction of the hair to create a line.

5. Triangle; square; rectangle; circle.

6. Yes, if the lotion is diluted with three times as much water.

7. No. Only a water soluble spray of very good quality should be used.

8. No. It is unsafe for the hair to be placed in hot dryers, and better sets will be obtained from longer drying times.

9. Slightly damp; heat rollers; hot irons.

10. Never roll sections of hair in a machine-made wig directly down a row or weft of hair.

11. A hairpiece styled into a geometric pattern of curls without any loose ends.

12. Clippies leave a mark on the hair.
13. This will produce smoother curls with more strength after drying.
14. Around the hairline or frame of the wig.
15. No.
16. No.

CHAPTER 7

1. The J and L Color Ring.
2. Processed hair is prepared by the factory for the color shades used on the different hair.
3. A temporary rinse that coats the hair and has no peroxide added.
4. A six-week color with no peroxide added.
5. Not at this time.
6. In order to set the color.
7. Yes.
8. An organic penetrating color.
9. Yes.
10. Lighter when wet; it will dry to a darker shade.
11. The nape area.
12. Detergent shampoo or stripping shampoo; stripper or stripper and peroxide; hair lightener and peroxide.
13. Yes, by metallic dye solvents.
14. No.

CHAPTER 8

1. Only human hair.
2. A method of permanent waving by using chemical solutions without heat.
3. The solution designed for bleached and porous or damaged hair.
4. To determine if the wig can be satisfactorily cold waved.
5. Curler size and thickness of hair strand.
6. Tension causes the hair to stretch, and the cold wave solution causes it to stretch even more, resulting in breakage and other serious damage.
7. When the process of wrapping the hair on the curlers is completed.
8. When, after unwinding the curler several turns, a strong letter "S" pattern is formed by the unrolled portion of the strand.

9. The time recommended by the manufacturer of the cold wave being used.
10. After completion of the cold waving process and before setting the style.
11. It discolors the hair, usually making it darker.

CHAPTER 9

1. Re-direction of curls; setting wigs, falls, and hairpieces; emergency sets and touchups.
2. Handle; spoon; and barrel.
3. Pin curls; roller curls; ridge waves.
4. Pre-heated curlers.
5. For quick sets and setting hair to do the put on of hairpieces.
6. A blower comb.
7. To blow dry and direct curl; to add body to hair; and to straighten over-curly synthetics.

CHAPTER 10

1. Three.
2. One for the customer; one for the hair left in service; and one for the wig stand or case left by the customer.
3. In case a question should arise pertaining to the customer's wig after she has left the salon.
4. Yes. So that there will not be any question as to the amount owed *after* you have completed your work.

CHAPTER 11

1. Selling is the link between the product and the need of the customer.
2. Without them you would have nothing to service and no clientele.
3. Because of the personal knowledge you must have about your customer and the fact that your judgment will guide the customer's decision.
4. A. Attitude. B. Greeting. C. Knowing the customer's needs. D. Price range. E. Showing the merchandise. F. Presentation of the merchandise. G. Answering questions about the merchandise. H. Customer selection. I. Ticket preparation. J. Follow-up on the sale.

CHAPTER 12

1. To satisfy yourself that the area will support the business.
2. In order to protect yourself by understanding the terms of the lease more fully.
3. From the State Cosmetology Commission at the state capital.
4. From the State Comptroller at the state capital.
5. It is required by law to cover your employees in the event of accidental injury while on the job.

CHAPTER 13

1. Applying single eyelashes to one's own natural lashes.
2. The synthetic lash; it has permanent curl and will not react to the weather.

CHAPTER 14

1. He could not compete with mass production.
2. Yes.
3. A V-shaped incision may be made to correct the fit.
4. In order to conform to the exact head shape.
5. A patch of false hair.
6. No. They vary in size according to the area of the head you want to cover.
7. Plastic wrap; masking tape.
8. In order to insure a better color match.
9. By spirit gum or tape.

GLOSSARY OF WIG TERMS

Affixative: Hair spray used to hold hair in its styled form.

Alura: Brand name of synthetic fiber sewn in wigs.

Antiseptic: Any substance that prevents the growth of bacteria.

Bacteria: Microscopic vegetable organisms, usually single-celled, multiplying by fission and spore formation.

Bailee liability: Insurance protection from loss of customer wigs.

Basting stitch: Loose stitch used in altering.

Bee's wax: Earliest affixative, comparable to lacquer or spraynet

Benzyl benzoate: Chemical used in treatment for contolling head lice.

Block: To fit wig onto canvas head.

Blocking: Fitting a wig on proper canvas head, following the customer's measurements.

Bulk: Thickness of hair

Canvas head: A canvas covered, cork-filled head used for setting, sizing, and blocking wigs.

Capless wig: Synthetic wig cap; wefts sewn on skeletal straps instead of solid material cap.

Chemical therapy: Treatment prescribed for people with cancer or tumors, resulting in loss of hair.

Cleaning solution, dry: A dry cleaning product in which wigs and hairpieces are cleaned

Cleaning solution, wet: A liquid cleaning product used on un-colored pieces or machine-made wigs

Coif: Cap that fits the head closely, such as a wig or a hairstyle

Coiffure: The style in which the hair is worn

Cold wave: Method of permanent waving using chemical waving and neutralizing solutions without the application of heat.

Cotton: Fiber generally used in making the caps of machine-made wigs.

Curl: A twist of hair forming a circle or semi-circle

Curler: Rod-type curler, usually of plastic, used in cold waving process

Customer: Your patron

Customer I. D. Card: Customer reference card containing head size, hair color, address, telephone number, hair samples, and other important information

Cutting down: Alteration by cutting sections from the wig cap

Darn: Mend a hole or tear in a wig cap by sewing back and forth

Dart: Flat seam used in altering

Disinfectant: Chemical means for preventing growth of bacteria

Dye solvents: Substance that removes artificial color from hair shaft

Elastic band: Band of elastic in back of a wig used in the sizing procedure

Elasticity: Having the quality of springing back to its original size or shape

Electric heat combs: Electric combs with heat and blower

European hair: Hair from European countries

Eye tabbing: The art of applying single artificial lashes

Eyelashes: Synthetic fiber eyelashes.

Fall: Longer hair, hairpiece

Fill in: To replace a few lashes

Filler: A style on a hairpiece that is used to fill-in or complete the hairstyle in a section of the head

First-quality hair: Hair cut from the head

Fitting: Alteration of a wig

Fumigants: Gas or fumes used in destroying germs

German white bleach: Bleaching compound used by wig manufacturers to bleach color from hair prior to tinting and assembling into finished hairpieces

Glue: Special adhesive used to apply the synthetic lashes

Goat hair: Yak hair used in making wigs for the very lightest white hair

Haircut: Shaping of hair into a precision form for a particular style

Hair goods: A general term applied to all wigs, hairpieces, and falls

Hair sample: Swatch of hair taken from patron's hair for matching purposes.

Hand-made (H.M. or H.T.):   A wig made by hand, the strands of hair being tied directly through the mesh cap and knotted on the outside of the cap. Also referred to as hand-tied or H.T.

Hand-tied (H.T.):   See Hand-made.

Heat rollers: Electric or steam pre-heated rollers

Hot irons: Instant curling method, using electric heat

International color ring: J & L Color Ring

J & L Color ring: The international color ring used to match your customer's hair in ordering a wig, hairpiece, or fall. This ring standardizes all the colors of the major manufacturers in the world of hair goods.

Kanekelon: Brand name of synthetic fiber sewn in wigs

Liability insurance: Protection from claims arising from accidental injuries on your premises

Machine-made (M.M.):   All machine-wefted wigs are totally machine-made.

Match test: Burning of fiber or hair to determine whether human or synthetic.

Maxi: Refers to longest lengths of hair

Measurements: Head size (around, front to back, ear to ear, temple to temple), necessary for sizing wigs

Midi: Refers to medium length hair

Mini: Refers to shortest lengths of hair

Natural hair: Unpermanented, uncolored hair

Neutralizer: Solution used in cold waving process to stop the action of the waving solution and re-harden the hair in a curled position around the curler

Normalizer: Solution used to acidify hair (usually one ounce vinegar to eight ounces water.

Nylon: Synthetic fiber used in making wigs, both in the cap and as hair

Occipital: Bone that forms the back part of the head

Operator: Term used for any person working on or with wigs and customers

Oriental hair: Hair from Asian countries such as China or Korea

Permanent color: Aniline-derivative tint, which when mixed with peroxide is a penetrating, permanent color

Permanent wave: Method of artificially forming waves or curls in hair, either by use of heat or chemicals, or both

Peruke: Wig (French)

Pick-up: Time designated by customer to pick-up, but not put-on, hair left in salon for service

Piece: Term used for all wigs or additional hair to be sold as hairgoods

Pin curl: Hair looped into circle to form a curl or wave

Porosity: Quality of hair to absorb moisture

Pre-cut: Factory-cut wigs

Processed hair: Finished hair (stripped, bleached, tinted, conditioned) ready to be sewn into wig

Processing: Manufacturing preparation of the hair prior to its being sewn into finished hairgoods (See Processed Hair)

Put-on: Placement of hairpiece or wig on a customer

Raw hair: Unprocessed hair

Reverse curl: Curl directioned away from the face

Sanitation: The practice of effecting healthful and hygienic conditions

Second-quality hair: Hair obtained from the combings of hair

Section: To part and separate the hair preparatory to coloring, cutting, or permanent waving

Semi-permanent rinse: A non-permanent color that coats and stains the hair, imparting color without peroxide

Semi-wig: Machine-made wig or hairpiece with front section hand-tied.

Silk: Material used in making the finer foundations for European handmade wigs

Sizing: Fitting or altering a wig to fit a person's head

Spirit gum: Glue used for attaching false hair

Sterilization: Process of freeing from living germs

Stretch base: Wig cap made of elastic materials that stretches from one size represented to fit all heads

Style: The specific size and shape of the finished wig or hairpiece, pertaining especially to the placement of curls, waves, bangs, and length.

Synthetic: Hairlike fibers, made by chemical synthesis, made into wigs and hairpieces.

Tape: Adhesive used to attach a patch of false hair

Tee pins: T-shaped pins used for blocking or holding rollers into place when setting

Test curls: Preliminary testing of the cold waving process on one or two curls to determine the advisability of cold waving the tested wig or hairpiece

Texture: Quality and structure of hair

Texturize: To thin

Thinning: Removing excess hair

Ticket system: Method of tagging customer pieces with instructions for required work

Toupee: A patch of false hair used to cover a bald spot

Try-on: A customer desiring to try a hairpiece or style

Tuck: Folded-over flat seam used in altering

Vegetable rinse: Temporary color rinse of organic origin

Venicelon: Brand name synthetic fiber sewn in wigs

Vise: Professional clamps that hold canvas blocks (while in use for styling or blocking wigs), attached to style bar or table

Weft: A machine-stitched strip of hair

Wholesaler: A representative that sells hairgoods to retailers

Wig: Artificial head covering of hair or synthetic fiber

Wig cap: The foundation that hair is attached to

Wig hamper: Bin designed to hold customer wigs that are in the salon for service

Wig industry: The manufacturers, wigologists, cosmotologists, retailers, and wholesalers who make, sell, and service wigs

Wigology: The study of wigs and artificial head coverings, including all phases of sales, service, and uses

Wig spray: A water-soluble, fine-mist, high-quality hairspray set

Workmen's compensation: The compensation to an employee for injury suffered in connection with his employment, paid under a government-supervised insurance system contributed to by employers

INDEX